THE PLAN

Shop, Stock and Serve.

Jessica Tinkler

iUniverse, Inc.
Bloomington

The Plan. Shop, Stock and Serve.

iUniverse books may be ordered through booksellers or by contacting:

iUniverse
1663 Liberty Drive
Bloomington, IN 47403
www.iuniverse.com
1-800-Authors (1-800-288-4677)

ISBN: 978-1-4502-9959-6 (pbk)
ISBN: 978-1-4502-9958-9 (ebk)

Printed in the United States of America

iUniverse rev. date: 4/5/11

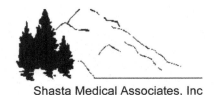

Shasta Medical Associates, Inc
www.shastamedical.com

MITCHELL S. AKMAN, MD, F.A.C.E.
BOARD CERTIFIED IN ENDOCRINOLOGY AND METABOLISM
FELLOW AMERICAN COLLEGE OF ENDOCRINOLOGY
BOARD CERTIFIED IN INTERNAL MEDICINE

As an endocrinologist, every day I see the devastating effects that poor lifestyle choices have on people's health. Complications of diabetes are the leading causes of blindness, kidney failure, and lower extremity nontraumatic amputations. Heart attacks and strokes are leading causes of morbidity and mortality in North America. Obesity and a sedentary life are two of the underlying root causes of these illnesses. In turn, all of these illnesses have their roots in lifestyle. However, as easy as it is to understand this concept, it is equally as difficult to do something about it. **The Plan** gives the reader a method for dealing with these issues head on. In clear and concise terms, Jessica gives systematic instructions on how to achieve a new, more appropriate and easily attainable healthy lifestyle. I have frequently told my patients that in order to be successful in managing their illnesses they need to plan ahead. This book puts that concept into writing and will give the reader the tools to be successful. I thoroughly enjoyed reading it and highly recommend it.

Mitchell S. Akman, M.D., Fellow of the American College of Endocrinologists

To my husband,
This book would never have been possible without his help, encouragement, love and support.

A note to the reader

There is strength in numbers. It is for that reason I encourage you to buy a friend a copy of this book. Having a friend will provide support, help, companionship and someone who can relate. Of course I must say, don't compete with each other- it's not a competition. Instead, help each other. Making lifestyle changes can be so much easier when you have someone along side you for support and who understands. Each week you will be able to lean on each other for the task at hand and help keep each other on track.

Disclaimer

I am not a doctor, I am an ordinary person. Much of this information stems from my own experiences. This book is designed to provide helpful information on subjects addressed. It is not intended to be a substitute for medical or psychological advice or counseling. You should consult a physician and/or mental health professional regarding your individual physical and mental heath needs before undertaking any lifestyle or diet change and/or fitness program. Keep in mind that diet and fitness recommendations will vary from person to person. I disclaim all liability associated with recommendations and guidelines set forth in this book. Please consider nutritional information as an estimate, it is not guaranteed to be 100% accurate.

Contents

Introduction

In life, without a PLAN, we don't know where to begin. We are always planning for our future, planning our vacation, planning our weekend. Making plans with friends (or we'd never see them). Making plans to visit family.

In order to get things done, everything needs some semblance of a PLAN.

THE PLAN is a very simple idea that will help you live a healthy lifestyle, while making sure it works within your lifestyle.

You PLAN your PLAN.

THE PLAN is not a diet; it's a way of living that fits into your world, not the other way around.

So, from here on out, I'm banning the phrase "going on a diet" from my brain (and yours too if you're up for it). I think you are because you're reading this book.

My hope for this book is that it provides you with the right tools so that the small changes you make will give you big results.

THE PLAN may seem very basic, because it is. Sometimes, the most obvious way to do things doesn't cross our minds. My job is to hit you over the head with it.

WHY THE PLAN WORKS:

*You won't have to make bad decisions in the heat of hunger anymore. The decision has already been made for you, by you!
*You don't have to worry about what's for dinner tonight. Or any meal or snack, for that matter.
*You will have healthy food already in the house.
*You eliminate that "crunch time" when you make unhealthy choices because you're famished.
*You have all the ingredients in your house to pack a lunch for work.
*You have a huge list of options, and lots of variety at your fingertips.

*You already have a snack set aside. When hunger hits, you don't have to go to the vending machine to fill a hole.

*Fewer trips to the grocery store means fewer chances of you picking up those last-minute bad food choices.

* THE PLAN is something you can realistically do for life.

What you put into your mouth directly affects how your body functions.[4-6] If you do already have Heart Disease[1,5], Type 2 Diabetes[2,5], or Hypertension[3,5] as a result of being overweight, *you* actually have the power to turn your diagnosis around![4,5] Putting the right foods into your body can literally change your health both inside and out. I'm really excited for you to start to see how these changes make you feel!

*You'll feel better about yourself.

*You'll be proud of yourself.

*You will gain a greater sense of self-esteem. [7]

*You'll get to fit into smaller sizes. Woo-hoo!

*You'll stop worrying about your weight and free that space in your brain for other things.

*You'll lower your risk of numerous diseases, including Coronary Artery Disease[1,5], Type 2 Diabetes[2,5], certain types of Cancers[5,8], Hypertension[3,5] and High Cholesterol[1,5], just to name a few. [5]

*You'll increase your life expectancy[6]. Isn't it nuts that food can actually do that?!

*You'll experience better moods and fewer mood swings. [7]

*You'll simply be more able to enjoy life!

Although your new lifestyle will directly affect your family (in a good way), you will be the one that feels majority of the benefits. It only makes sense that THE PLAN focuses on you. THE PLAN demands that you take time to treat yourself with care, love, respect and honesty. For some of us, this could be a first.

Here is the first step:

Hey, Sweet Sixteen! We're Keeping a Diary!

Before you begin your new outlook on healthy living, you must evaluate your old one. In order to understand why you're currently looking to lose weight now, you need to fully grasp how you have been living and what got you here. Remember, food is a choice. A diary forces you to make it a conscious one.

Starting right now (life does not begin tomorrow, nor does it begin on Monday), continue to live and eat the way you normally do. However, I want you to document every single thing you eat and drink for seven days. I mean everything. The only way this is going to work is if you write it *all* down. And please, be honest with yourself. This can be a tough evaluation for some. It can be a good, honest and hard look in the mirror. Even if you try the sample frappaccino at Starbucks, <u>put it in the diary</u>. One piece of gum, one carrot stick, one Tic Tac, one ounce sample—it all goes in your diary. The diary is the first step toward your new outlook.

I had a client once who recorded her one-week food diary for me, very diligently I might add. Before we sat down to discuss it, she handed the diary over to me and said, *"I know, I know, I should not have had three slices of pizza on Thursday and the ice cream on Tuesday night was really bad. I know! Oh, and I like my wine. I know I drink too much."*

The purpose of the diary is not to point out all the things you should not have eaten. We all know that a bag of chips is bad for us. What I want the diary to do is be able to highlight all the good choices you are making and lay out the small, subtle things you can do gradually that will make the difference!

On that note!

<u>BUY A PAD TO KEEP TRACK!!</u>

Buy a small pad and carry it with you throughout the day. Every time you eat something (be it a beverage or a sandwich), take out your diary and write it down. Please, pretty please, I beg you: Do not wait until the end of the day to do this. It defeats the purpose. You may say you won't forget, but you will. That bag of Goldfish you shared with your two-year-old will be forgotten as well as the half-bottle of Diet Coke. Oh, and that handful of Doritos: Did I have just one handful? Crap, I had that apple too!

Record:
Time:
What you ate:
How much you ate:
Beverages: including water

Here is an example of a day in the life:

7am - Coffee w̄ milk - 2 cups

10am - 1 bagel w̄ cream cheese. ~~Banana~~ 1 banana.

11:30 am - Bag of chips, Diet coke.

12:15 - 3 twizzlers (at office)

1:30 - Subway Sub 12" w̄ assorted meat, cheese, mayo
       + Diet coke

4:00 - Apple

6:00 - Triscuit (crackers) - Maybe 15

7:00 - Chick. Breast w̄ BBQ sauce, Baked potatoe w̄
       sour cream + chive, Uncle Bens Rice w̄ veggie (Peas & carrots),
       green beans

8:00 pm - Couple spoonfuls of rice (from dinner)

8:30 - Bag of microwave Popcorn (shared w̄ wife)

9:45 - 2 oreo cookies - sm. glass of milk.

You may find it a pain to carry around a diary and record everything as you eat it- but it's only a week: seven days! Or, you may love the insight it provides you. You can diary every week if you want! In fact, I find using a diet diary is a huge step toward success! In fact, if you are fortunate enough to have a buddy reading this book with you, I encourage you to email each other your diet diaries at the end of the day. This way you are accountable to someone other than yourself.

As you read along, you will learn little tips and tricks that will help you identify your old habits. You'll be able to look back at your diary and see where you have made the small changes you can live with. You shouldn't feel cheated because you want to live a healthy life.

Feel free to use this template. There are more at the back of the book.

Diet Diary

7.00 am-

8.00 am-

9.00 am-

10.00 am-

11.00 am-

12.00 pm-

1.00 pm-

2.00 pm-

3.00 pm-

4.00 pm-

5.00 pm-

6.00 pm-

7.00 pm-

8.00 pm-

9.00 pm-

10.00 pm-

11.00 pm-

12.00 am-

1.00 am-

Now that you have your seven-day diary and you know where you are coming from, you're ready to start PLANNING for your future! This is the best part.

"Today is a new day!"

It doesn't matter what happened yesterday. It's in the past. It will not affect how you live today, <u>if you don't let it</u>. Let yesterday be forgotten and look forward from today. Do this every day!

If you have not already done so:

Step on a scale.
(First thing in the AM after your morning pee)
Let's face it. We want to see the lowest, most consistent number ☺

Measure your waist.
(Suck in and measure around your bellybutton. You'll always remember where you measured from and I know you'll always suck in. Consistency is key!)

Record it.

These numbers are merely benchmarks for you. Today, it does not matter where you are compared to the rest of the world. Where you are now is where you are. Period. The fact that you're still reading this book means you're looking to make some kind of change. If you stick with THE PLAN, the number on your scale can only go down. Your waist circumference can only shrink. When you check back with yourself in a couple of weeks you will have new numbers to compare with your old ones.

20 Reasons!

I want you to list 20 reasons why you want to lose the weight. Yes, 20. Whether you have 10 pounds to lose or 200 pounds. When you think you cannot think of any more reasons, get creative!

Ask yourself...

How are you living now?   How do you want to live?

Who are you losing the weight for?
Yourself?   Your family?   Your future?
Why?
To fit into your favorite jeans?   Your doctor said you should?

I'm asking you and I will continue to ask you throughout this journey to be honest with yourself. No one is going to see this list but you. Even if it scares you to write it down, write it. Make it real for yourself. Even if you think it's a silly reason, it's all relative. These reasons belong to you and they are important because they are yours.

1. ....

2. ....

3. ....

4. ....

5. ....

6. ....

7. ....

8. ....

9. ....

10. ....

11. ....

12. ....

13. ....

14. ....

15. ....

16. ....

17. ....

18. ....

19. ....

20. ....

I once read an article written by a psychologist that really struck a chord with me. It read something to the effect of:

> *"People that want to lose weight but still say yes to the dessert or the second helpings <u>don't actually, really care</u> about losing weight. It's simply <u>not that important</u> to them"*

Now you have 20 reasons why it is important to you.

The Contract

Take a blank piece of paper, have a seat with a nice cup of tea and talk to yourself. Write yourself a letter. _With love_. This is not a beat-myself-up free-for-all. Tell yourself why you deserve to be healthy and happy from the inside out. Why this time is _the_ time you're going to make the changes that stick. And know that you are 100% capable of doing it.

We are so hard on ourselves; no wonder we set ourselves up for failure. If you consistently had a friend or a lover telling you "Your pants don't fit, why did you eat that? You idiot, look at that jiggle hanging from your arms!" you would hate that person. But we do it to ourselves every day for some strange reason!

You need to be your own best friend here, not your worst enemy.

Write this letter to yourself, date it and at the very end, make a promise to yourself. Tell yourself all the positive things you are going to do to start taking care of your body. It's up to you to live the rest of your life the way you truly want to live it: happy, healthy, confident and strong. One day at a time, please.

Whether it's:
Get off my meds   Eat three healthy meals a day
Stop night binging
Stop obsessing about food   Be free of dieting
Love myself again   Take time for myself
Think positive thoughts

Whatever it is, write it down! There is no wrong way to write a letter to yourself! Then, sign it. Keep this letter in a safe place. If there comes a time where you start to slip, you can always come back to this letter and to your 20 reasons.

One more piece of business and we are ready to roll!

Back to Basics

There is no secret trick to losing weight. You just have to find a way of losing weight that you can live with. Before we get to THE PLAN, I want you to understand the nuts and bolts of all weight loss programs.

The truth is, all weight loss plans focus on lowering your calorie intake. In order to lose weight, you have to eat fewer calories than you are using up. [9, 10]

Here is the dirt on losing a pound:
* Studies suggest one pound is equivalent to approximately 3500 calories. [11]
* In order to lose body fat you need to eat fewer calories than you use. [9, 12-15]
* In order to lose one pound you need to cut approximately 3500 calories. [9-15, 17]

How?
If you cut 500 calories a day, you will lose one pound a week. [9-15]

or

If you cut 250 calories a day and burn 250 calories with exercise you will also lose one pound a week. [9-15]

Everyone has a number of calories they need in a day. These calories keep their organs functioning, their blood flowing and their body temperature regulated. This is called your Resting Metabolic Rate or RMR.

How do you know the number of calories you need?

There are medical tests that can be done to supply you with your precise number. For the purpose of this book I have provided an equation that will give you an estimate as to how many calories you need in a day.

This is a general formula. It is not specific to how much lean muscle mass you have. The more muscle you have, the more efficient your metabolism, the more calories you need!

Mifflin Equation [16, 17]

MEN:
    RMR= (9.99 x your weight in kg) + (6.25 x your height in cm) − (4.92 x your age) + 5

<u>WOMEN:</u>

RMR= (9.99 x your weight in kg) + (6.25 x your height in cm) – (4.92 x your age) -161

- your weight in kg = your weight in lbs divided by 2.2
- your height in cm = your height in inches multiplied by 2.54

Now multiply your answer by your activity level:

Sedentary: 1.200 (little to no exercise)
Lightly Active: 1.375 (light exercise, sports, 1-3 days a week)
Moderately Active: 1.550 (moderate exercise sports, 3-5 days a week)
Very Active: 1.725 (hard exercise, sports, 6-7 days a week)
Extra Active: 1.900 (very hard daily exercise and sports, very physical job)

My example-
I am 105 lbs = 105 divided by 2.2 = 47.727 kg
I am 62 inches tall = 62 inches multiplied by 2.54 =   157.48 cm

I am 31
(9.99 x 47.727) + (6.25 x 157.48) – (4.92 x 31) -161
   (476.792) +   (984.25) –   (152.52) - 161=   1147.522

1147.522 x 1.550 (active) = 1778.66

To lose one pound a week: 1778.66 – 500 = 1278

I could eat 1278 calories a day. ***OR***
I could eat 1528 calories a day, and burn 250 calories a day with exercise.

Now you have the tools that will show you approximately how many calories you need to subtract with food and how many calories you can choose to burn through exercise.

It's a good idea to know your number, if even just to keep it in the back of your mind. As you begin to read labels and look at portions you will have a better idea of how things fit into your day. If you follow the steps of THE PLAN, you should be able to live without having to count calories every day. But if you want to count your calories, feel free to do so. It can be very helpful.

*I strongly DO NOT recommend going lower than 1200[18] calories a day. With anything less than 1200 calories a day your body believes it is starving. Your body becomes afraid that it won't get any more food, and as a result it will hold onto the little amount of food you are eating and store it. This will prevent you from losing weight; you may even gain weight. [19, 20] **You have to fuel your body to lose weight; starving yourself is not the answer.**

*As you lose weight, the number of calories you need in a day will change.
Make sure that every time you have a weigh-in, you have a second look at this equation

Alrighty, enough of the math! Here comes THE PLAN!

*Don't conquer the world in a day. Change takes time. Be
generous with yourself and give yourself the time.*

Small changes make a lifetime of difference. Trust me, the slower you go, the more it sticks. You
can't conquer Rome in a day and anyone that tells you otherwise is lying. Be easy on yourself (to
an extent). Whether you have five or 150 pounds to lose, you sure didn't gain the weight in a day,
so don't try to lose it all in a day either. The more time you give yourself the more likely you are
to stick with a healthy lifestyle and keep the weight off.

THE PLAN is simple. PLAN your week! That's it.

The Plan

Plan out your meals, then ***shop, stock and serve***!

- — Make a list of easy breakfast, lunch and dinner ideas.
- — Make a list of quick and delicious snack ideas.
- — Write a grocery list based on your meal and snack ideas.
- — ***Shop, stock and serve!***

Okay, let's all be honest here. It would be nice to think we cook something new every day, but who does that? I'm no Martha Stewart. Most of us find our favorite foods and we stick to them. Every morning I have one of two things for breakfast. Rarely do I veer. For sure, I barbeque chicken <u>at least</u> twice a week. My lunches are either leftovers from dinner or one of my go-tos (of which I have *maybe* three). We all fall into our habits, and that's 100% okay. Use your habits! Having habits makes eating healthy so much easier to stick to. Having said that, it's okay to repeat meals on your MASTER PLAN. You can have the same thing for breakfast every day if you want to! But writing it down gives you direction and you're less likely to find yourself off course.

The *Recipe and Ideas* section of this book, as well as *My Favorite Foods*, is made up of many of my habits. It's the way I try to cook and eat at home, and the way I snack.

Your PLAN is just as important as exercise. On the day you make your MASTER PLAN, make it your healthy living priority. If you can't find time to exercise on this day, that's 100% okay. Your "exercise" time was the 15 minutes you took for yourself to make your PLAN, bettering yourself from the inside out! Having a PLAN will give you a great healthy launching pad for your coming week.

HOW TO MAKE YOUR MASTER PLAN:

The night before you do your grocery shopping, sit down and chart out what you are going to eat for breakfast, lunch, dinner and your snacks for the next week. Have a look in your fridge and freezer to see what you already have in the house. Make a grocery list based on the ingredients you will need to make *all* the meals on your MASTER PLAN.

Do you ever come home from the grocery store having spent 50 or 100 dollars on food, look in your fridge and can't seem to put a decent meal together? The broccoli you bought (with the best intentions) goes bad. The fish you purchased now has freezer burn and the healthy yogurt you wanted to try expired before you had a chance to open it. Now, you are shopping with a purpose! You are buying foods specific to the meals you are PLANNING to make. Your fruits and vegetables won't go bad in the veggie drawer any more.

To help you with ideas of good food choices to include on your MASTER PLAN, check out the *My Favorite Foods* section. If you're looking for easy meal and snacks, have a browse through the recipe portion of this book. Get out a highlighter and highlight the recipes you would like to try.

On your MASTER PLAN write down one or two recipes or ideas you would like to try and a few of your tried and true favorites. Don't forget that whatever you cook for dinner, you'll probably have leftovers for the next day's lunch. Put leftovers on your PLAN. And of course, repeat meals and snacks as much as you like.

Write your grocery list based on your MASTER PLAN and hit the Market!

This means you only have to shop <u>once a week </u>(except maybe for milk)! You'll be fully stocked to try a couple of new healthy recipes and a couple of old favorites!

*If you have kids and you pack a lunch for them, try to PLAN out their lunches so that you can put what you need on your grocery list. You'll still get all your shopping done in one visit.

WHAT MY MASTER PLAN LOOKS LIKE:

MONDAY

Breakfast: Fresh Fruit + ~~Oatmeal (Banana)~~

Snack: ↓ Oatmeal w̄ banana

Lunch: Turkey Sandwich

Snack: cheese string

Dinner: Grilled chicken w̄ salad

TUESDAY

Breakfast: Fresh Fruit + ~~oatmeal (Ban)~~

Snack: ↓ Oatmeal w̄ banana

Lunch: left over chicken in wrap

Snack: milk w̄ chocolate milk

Dinner: Salmon w̄ easy couscous

WEDNESDAY

Breakfast: Fresh Fruit ~~oatmeal (Ban)~~

Snack: ↓ oatmeal w̄ banana

Lunch: couscous leftovs

Snack: Frozen yogurt

Dinner: Baked Chicken Parm + Asparagus

THURSDAY

Breakfast: Cereal w̄ milk

Snack: cottage cheese ~~berries~~

Lunch: Peanut Butter + banana sandwich

Snack: 1oz cashews

Dinner: Quiche w̄ quinoa.

FRIDAY

Breakfast: Fruit

Snack: Breakfast cookie

Lunch: ~~Toast on celery~~ Quiche left over + quinoa.

Snack: cheese string

Dinner: No Noodle lasagna w̄ ceasar salad.

SATURDAY

Breakfast: Yogurt w̄ Berries

Snack: Apple + Parm cheese

Lunch: ~~Tuna Salad on celery~~ left over lasagna.

Snack: → not going to have as I am going for early dinner

Dinner: Going out for Dinner (will order fish w̄ veg.. 1 glass wine + 1 peice bread).

SUNDAY

Breakfast: meeting friends for brunch

Snack: → Brunch (egg white omlete + WW toast).

Lunch: → Brunch

Snack: ½ Lara Cashew Bar.

Dinner: Making Pizza at home on whole wheat crust.

WHAT MY GROCERY LIST LOOKS LIKE:

GROCERY LIST

Fruits and Veggies:
Berries
lettuce
Asparagus
veggies for Pizza-
Spinach + mush for quiche (and lasagna)
bananas
cottage cheese
zuchini
celry
Baby carrots
cucumber

Whole Grains (Cereals, Breads, Rice ect..):
sprouted grain
cous cous
quinoa
whole grain pizza dough
wraps (Sonoma if thy have it).

Dairy (Cheese, Eggs, Yogurt, Milk, ect..):
chase strings   ricotta cheese
parmesan
milk
Eggs

Dips, Sauces & Spices:
peanut butter.
tomato sauce

Have in house
Kiwi
Apple
grapefruit
Banana's - need more.
Oatmeal
Chicken
chocolate milk
yogurt
cottage cheese - need more
Asiago
mozzarella 2%.

Meats and Fish:
Salmon
turkey sausage.
turky Bacon (wrap + cesar salad)

Other :

So far, we are spending 15 minutes one night a week PLANNING out our meals, snacks and making a grocery list!

DAILY MAINTENANCE

Now on Wednesday night, if you don't feel like eating the salmon you've put on your PLAN, you don't have to have it.

Your fridge is full of healthy meal options for you to choose from.

Maybe you feel like eating the steak you have in your freezer that you were PLANNING on eating Friday night! The point is, you have healthy and easy meal ideas already laid out. You don't have to struggle to think of something to eat, and in frustration, end up with take-out. Look at your Master Plan. **Think of it as a menu!** What else is on there that piques your taste buds? Have that instead! You already have all the ingredients in your house to make it.

Every night:
Take five minutes for yourself. Have a look-see at your Master Plan and PLAN out your next day.

Remember that the Master Plan you created at the beginning of the week is flexible. Just follow your taste buds! Rarely do I eat what I have PLANNED out for my next day. I normally end up eating what I was going to eat Tuesday on Friday and the snack that I put down on Sunday ends up in my mouth on Monday. Don't ever feel like you have to eat what you have written down for the next day. Please feel free to switch it up!

Decide what you want the next day for your breakfast, lunch, dinner and your two snacks.

Take whatever you need out of the freezer to prepare for tomorrow's dinner, marinate your meat, or do whatever preparatory steps you can to make dinner easy and simple when you get home from work. Take five minutes, and then make your lunch and pack your snacks. You're good to go!

I have put together examples of my Tuesday and Wednesday for you:

Tuesday

DAILY PLAN

Breakfast: Cereal + milk (shredded bit size mini wheats).

Snack: apple

Lunch: left over chicken in Ceaser wrap.

Snack: Cashews (1 oz)

Dinner: Salmon w̄ couscous.
→ Just made couscous plain w̄ chicken soup broth some almonds + dried herbs.

Wednesday

DAILY PLAN

Breakfast: Fruit (Kiwi, apple ½) grapefruit ½

Snack: oatmeal w̄ ½ banana.

Lunch: left over Salmon w̄ couscous
→ ended up saving salmon fa Thursday lunch + having a Peanut Butter + Banana sandwich w̄ milk.

Snack: nope

Dinner: No Noodle lasagna.
Try not to eat later than. — went out at 8:15 fa
Treat! Around 8pm - Frozen yogurt. out for. → yogurt. not bad

Other things to consider when making your PLAN.

This is your PLAN. You get to decide how and what you're going to eat. Just because the template has three meals and two snacks a day does not mean you *have* to eat this way. If a different way of dividing up your meals works for you, cool, go for it!

What kind of eater are you?

Identify and work within your boundaries. Don't try to become a whole new person. Work with what you've got!

Do you like…
<u>Big Portions?</u> Then make sure your plate is filled with greenery! This will allow you to still enjoy big filling plates of food without the extra calories.

Are you a…
<u>Snacker?</u> Why not make your three meals and two snacks into six or even seven. This is what I do! I have:

1) First breakfast
2) Second breakfast
3) Snack
4) Lunch
5) Snack
6) Dinner

I make my meals a bit smaller so that I can eat more often.

Can we just admit that we are….
<u>Lazy:</u> Well if this is you, I have over 100 ideas in the recipe section for easy, healthy and fast breakfasts, lunches, dinners and snacks. You just have to PLAN ahead. Do your grocery shopping once a week and have it all in the house.

A lot of us just do it because we have nothing better to do. We're…
<u>Bored Eaters</u>: A great way to overcome this to come up with ideas that will help you get through the hard times. Decaf or flavored hot tea, water, painting your nails, reading or emailing a friend are great ways to keep your hands and mouths occupied! I know these are much easier said then done, but sometimes healthy eating is just as much about our minds as it is or tummies. Write a list for yourself of things you can do when you're bored. Post it on your fridge. Read it before you open the door.
I will talk about treats, eating out and alcoholic beverages; that all starts in *"Life's Little Curve Balls"*! But fret not, you can put them all on your PLAN! In fact, whatever you want to eat can go on your PLAN.

Week One On The Plan

Just Add Water

Take this week to simply get used to the PLAN and add some good old water.

Focus on laying out your week. Get used to the idea of coming up with easy meal ideas and packing your house with healthy foods. Again, you can use the Recipe and Meal Ideas at the back of this book for any help you need.

The one other thing that gets included in your daily activity is my very favorite life tip!

1. *PEE CLEAR*

Water is nature's weight loss remedy! Buy yourself a one-liter bottle of water and fill and finish it at least two times a day. [21] Become one with your pee! Have a look in the potty; if your pee is not clear or pale yellow, you need more water!

*For those of you taking a multi-vitamin, as your body flushes what it does not need, your pee becomes fluorescent yellow/orange. [22] It is very simple to distinguish a "vitamin pee" from a "non-hydrated" one. The urine from your vitamins has a very distinct color. If you properly hydrate, fluorescent yellow will turn to a pale yellow or clear throughout the day.

<u>Why water is so darn good</u>
Everyone tells you to drink it, now you'll know why!

Did you know?

*When most people begin to feel the onset of hunger they are actually simply thirsty. Drinking water can prevent you from eating that extra snack. Water suppresses your appetite![23, 25] Water is food! This may not be the most fun thing to learn, since popcorn tends to taste much better than water. But would you fill your car's gas tank if you just needed windshield washer fluid? No. Eat the right food for the right job. Your body will thank you.

*Water is a key to your body metabolizing fat. With enough water, your metabolism will work more efficiently to burn fat as fuel. [24]

*When your body does not get enough water, it will begin to hold onto every drop. This causes fluid retention and bloating. The more water you drink, the less you will retain, and the less you will bloat. [24, 25]

*Water helps your body rid itself of unneeded salt, which can be a major factor in high blood pressure. [25]

*Water helps rid your body of waste[25] (fat is waste). During weight loss, your body has a lot more waste to get rid of; fat must be shed and water must be present to help your system get it done. [24, 25]

*A little water can go a long way when it comes to your stool. When your body gets too little water from outside sources, it takes it from the inside (the colon is one of the primary places it gets it) and this causes constipation. [24, 25]

Water Can Also: [24, 25]
Boost energy levels
Alleviate some headaches
Help to reduce blood pressure
Help to reduce high cholesterol

It is possible, but very unlikely that you will drink too much water. Here is a guideline you can follow:

*You should consume two to three liters of water a day. [23]
*For weight loss, you should consume one additional eight-ounce glass for every 25 pounds you are overweight. [23]

MORAL OF THE STORY : A healthy pee is a clear one!

THIS WEEK

FOLLOW YOUR PLAN
PEE CLEAR

* Tips
- Get together or phone a friend to help map out your Master Plan this week.
- Feel free to check in with each other to see how the water intake is going.

YOUR WEEK ONE WORKSHEET AND GROCERY LIST:

MONDAY

Breakfast:

Snack:

Lunch:

Snack:

Dinner:

TUESDAY

Breakfast:

Snack:

Lunch:

Snack:

Dinner:

WEDNESDAY

Breakfast:

Snack:

Lunch:

Snack:

Dinner:

THURSDAY

Breakfast:

Snack:

Lunch:

Snack:

Dinner:

FRIDAY

Breakfast:

Snack:

Lunch:

Snack:

Dinner:

SATURDAY

Breakfast:

Snack:

Lunch:

Snack:

Dinner:

SUNDAY

Breakfast: Lunch: Dinner:

Snack: Snack:

GROCERY LIST

Fruits and Veggies:

Whole Grains (Cereals, Breads, Rice ect..):

Dairy (Cheese, Eggs, Yogurt, Milk, ect..) :

Dips, Sauces & Spices:

Meats and Fish:

Other :

DAILY PLAN

Breakfast:

Snack:

Lunch:

Snack:

Dinner:

DAILY PLAN

Breakfast:

Snack:

Lunch:

Snack:

Dinner:

DAILY PLAN

Breakfast:

Snack:

Lunch:

Snack:

Dinner:

DAILY PLAN

Breakfast:

Snack:

Lunch:

Snack:

Dinner:

DAILY PLAN

Breakfast:

Snack:

Lunch:

Snack:

Dinner:

DAILY PLAN

Breakfast:

Snack:

Lunch:

Snack:

Dinner:

DAILY PLAN

Breakfast:

Snack:

Lunch:

Snack:

Dinner:

DAILY PLAN

Breakfast:

Snack:

Lunch:

Snack:

Dinner:

Week Two On The Plan

Congrats on completing week one! We're on the way! This week we are going to add what I believe to be the most important step. It's actually the one that takes the most practice. Do your best to keep mindful of these tips. We are not all perfect, we all make mistakes, but as you start to make these changes, they will begin to become easier for you to do. Take your time. Don't beat yourself up and for goodness' sake. Have some fun with it!

WE ARE ALREADY….

MAKING A PLAN
PEEING CLEAR

WE ARE NOW ADDING *Portion Control* to the mix!

1. PORTION CONTROL[25]
No matter how healthy you eat, too much of anything is too much.

This week:
    Learn your portions

Almost everything you eat will come with labels. It is very important to read and follow the serving sizes on the label. Pay close attention to how much a serving size is, and how many servings are in the box. Most people assume a huge muffin is one serving, but most of the time it's actually two.

Pour your morning bowl of cereal into a measuring cup before you pour it into your bowl. Look at your labels. They are there for a reason, I swear!

If you want ice cream as one of your snacks this week, have it. One serving of ice cream **(½ cup)** never hurt anyone.

Take this time to learn what your portions look like on your plates and in your bowls at home. Once you have a feel for how your portions look, you can stop measuring. But, be diligent. Every once and a while, come back to measuring your portions. Just check in with yourself to make sure your eyes didn't start playing tricks on you.

PASTA: [26] Normally you're looking at about three-fourths of a cup or two ounces. But check the label of the brand you buy. Measure it out a couple of times so you can see how many noodles you get to eat in relation to your bowl at home. Then fill out your pasta with veggies and protein! The bowl gets pretty full, pretty quickly.

PROTEIN: [27] One serving of protein is 3-4 ounces. I recommend:
    3-4 ounces for women
    6 ounces for men

I measure my protein on a kitchen scale once it's been cooked.

A cheap scale at your local kitchen store should run you $10-15. It's a worthwhile investment that you should make if you can.

FRUIT: [27] They say compare your apple to a baseball—kind of tough to do. All apples look like the size of baseballs to me. This is where your scale comes into play. But if you don't have a scale on hand:

Typically, round fruit is approximately 2-3 inches in diameter per serving.
Bananas should be no more than 6 inches long or 3.5 ounces per serving.

Grapefruit	½ of the fruit
Berries	½ cup
Dried Fruit	¼ cup
Avocado	1 ounce (3 slices)

VEGETABLES: I personally (although, some would disagree) don't think you can have too many green vegetables, especially if you're someone who likes a big plate of food. Have as many servings of green vegetables as you like (as long as they are not covered in butter!).

When the color is not green, have a closer look at your serving size. [27]

Sweet Potato	½ cup mashed
Carrots	3 ounces (that's about 15 baby carrots)
Squash	½ cup
Potato	½ cup (normally half a potato)
Corn	An ear 5-6 inches long/1/3 cup niblets

NUTS: Approximately 1 ounce [26, 27]

23 almonds	18 Cashew Nuts	7 Brazil Nuts	7 walnuts

I know this is a lot of information. And this is where you will make the most changes. But I'm not asking you to stop eating the pasta or the ice cream. I'm asking you to just look at how much you are eating.

A good way to stop yourself from having more than your portion's worth:

Rate your hunger on a scale of 1-10.
Stop eating at around a **7 out of 10.**

If you stop and have some water, you'll fill up much faster. Don't wait until you feel full to have water. Stop. Drink water.

It's not a lie when nutritionists tell you that it takes 20 minutes for your body to signal to your brain that you've had enough food. I don't know about you, but I can eat a bowl of cereal in less than three minutes! If you think you may still be hungry, have a glass of good old H20 to top you up, wait 20 minutes and see how you feel.

I know it's not the easiest thing to say, "I'll only have a half-cup of my very favorite ice cream and stop at that." Moderation and portion control can be a challenge. They take time. Give yourself that! Practice! One of my favorite mantras is:

"I want to learn the practice of moderation, in moderation."

Until you are certain you can practice moderation with the foods you tend to go overboard on, don't put them on your PLAN just yet. Once you have built up some strength and courage, give it a try. If it works, great! Put your favorites on the PLAN. If not, try and try again.

How often can you put treats on your PLAN?
Well, that's entirely up to you! Try putting them on once every three days to start. See how that works for you. I have some clients that like to have one treat a week so that they feel like it's really a treat. I have other clients that like to have one of their snacks as a 100 or 150 calorie treat everyday so that they never feel deprived.

THIS WEEK
FOLLOW YOUR PLAN

PEE CLEAR

WATCH YOUR PORTIONS
(7 out of 10)

*Tips
- Use your week one MASTER PLAN to help you map out week two.
- Repeat your favorites from the week and try 1 or 2 new ideas.
- Get together or phone a friend! Call each other when you have questions about portions or when you've found a great new snack you love!

YOUR WEEK TWO WORKSHEET AND GROCERY LIST:

MONDAY

Breakfast:

Snack:

Lunch:

Snack:

Dinner:

TUESDAY

Breakfast:

Snack:

Lunch:

Snack:

Dinner:

WEDNESDAY

Breakfast:

Snack:

Lunch:

Snack:

Dinner:

THURSDAY

Breakfast:

Snack:

Lunch:

Snack:

Dinner:

FRIDAY

Breakfast:

Snack:

Lunch:

Snack:

Dinner:

SATURDAY

Breakfast:

Snack:

Lunch:

Snack:

Dinner:

SUNDAY

Breakfast: Lunch: Dinner:

Snack: Snack:

GROCERY LIST

Fruits and Veggies:

Whole Grains (Cereals, Breads, Rice ect..):

Dairy (Cheese, Eggs, Yogurt, Milk, ect..) :

Dips, Sauces & Spices:

Meats and Fish:

Other :

DAILY PLAN

Breakfast:

Snack:

Lunch:

Snack:

Dinner:

DAILY PLAN

Breakfast:

Snack:

Lunch:

Snack:

Dinner:

DAILY PLAN

Breakfast:

Snack:

Lunch:

Snack:

Dinner:

DAILY PLAN

Breakfast:

Snack:

Lunch:

Snack:

Dinner:

DAILY PLAN

Breakfast:

Snack:

Lunch:

Snack:

Dinner:

DAILY PLAN

Breakfast:

Snack:

Lunch:

Snack:

Dinner:

DAILY PLAN

Breakfast:

Snack:

Lunch:

Snack:

Dinner:

DAILY PLAN

Breakfast:

Snack:

Lunch:

Snack:

Dinner:

Week Three On The Plan

We are already - **MAKING A PLAN**
- **PEEING CLEAR**
- **WATCHING OUR PORTIONS (7 out of 10)**

WE ARE NOW ADDING Getting at least *25 grams of fiber* a day. [28, 30]

You've now mastered reading labels, so read 'em till you reach the number 25 on your fiber count. Add up those grams of fiber!

Everyone tells you to eat it, and now you'll know why!

Fun Fact about Fiber: Fiber is the part of the plant or the grain that humans can't digest. It's actually calorie free. [29]

Insoluble Fiber:

*It soaks up water much like a sponge and adds a bulkiness and softness to your stool. [28]

*It not only prevents constipation and reduces hemorrhoid risk but also reduces the rate at which food goes through your system and colon. This type of fiber helps you feel fuller—great for weight loss! [28]

Foods high in insoluble fiber: [29]
Whole-wheat flour   Bran   Vegetables   Whole grains
Fruits with edible seeds such as strawberries

Soluble Fiber:

*This type of fiber forms a gel-like substance in water. [29]
  (It's what gives oatmeal its gummy texture)

*As it passes through the digestive system, soluble fiber binds to dietary cholesterol, helping the body eliminate it, aiding in the prevention of heart disease and stroke. [28] I really think it's amazing that food is capable of doing these great things for our bodies!

*Soluble fiber slows glucose digestion, helping to control diabetes. [28]

*Also aids in constipation, holding moisture in your stool to soften it. [28]

Food high in soluble fiber: [29]
Oats   Legumes   Barley   Apples
Citrus fruits   Strawberries   Carrots

THIS WEEK
FOLLOW YOUR PLAN

PEE CLEAR

WACTH YOUR PORTIONS
*(7 out of 10)

25 GRAMS OF FIBER

*Tips
- Use your week two MASTER PLAN to help you map out week three.
- Repeat your favorites from the week and try one or two fiber-rich ideas.
- Get together or phone a friend! When you find something high in fiber, share the news!

YOUR WEEK THREE WORKSHEET AND GROCERY LIST:

MONDAY

Breakfast:

Snack:

Lunch:

Snack:

Dinner:

TUESDAY

Breakfast:

Snack:

Lunch:

Snack:

Dinner:

WEDNESDAY

Breakfast:

Snack:

Lunch:

Snack:

Dinner:

THURSDAY

Breakfast:

Snack:

Lunch:

Snack:

Dinner:

FRIDAY

Breakfast:

Snack:

Lunch:

Snack:

Dinner:

SATURDAY

Breakfast:

Snack:

Lunch:

Snack:

Dinner:

SUNDAY

Breakfast: Lunch: Dinner:

Snack: Snack:

GROCERY LIST

Fruits and Veggies:

Whole Grains (Cereals, Breads, Rice ect..):

Dairy (Cheese, Eggs, Yogurt, Milk, ect..) :

Dips, Sauces & Spices:

Meats and Fish:

Other :

DAILY PLAN

Breakfast:

Snack:

Lunch:

Snack:

Dinner:

DAILY PLAN

Breakfast:

Snack:

Lunch:

Snack:

Dinner:

DAILY PLAN

Breakfast:

Snack:

Lunch:

Snack:

Dinner:

DAILY PLAN

Breakfast:

Snack:

Lunch:

Snack:

Dinner:

DAILY PLAN

Breakfast:

Snack:

Lunch:

Snack:

Dinner:

DAILY PLAN

Breakfast:

Snack:

Lunch:

Snack:

Dinner:

DAILY PLAN

Breakfast:

Snack:

Lunch:

Snack:

Dinner:

DAILY PLAN

Breakfast:

Snack:

Lunch:

Snack:

Dinner:

Week Four On The Plan

We are already - **MAKING A PLAN**
                 - **PEEING CLEAR**
                 - **WATCHING OUR PROTIONS (7 out of 10)**
                 - **GETTING 25 GRAMS OF FIBER A DAY**

WE ARE NOW ADDING *Closing the kitchen two hours before bed*.

If you're not sure if you're going to bed at 10:00 pm or 11:30 pm, just stop at 8:00pm.

Always start and end your day with water.

After a healthy dinner, your body does not need more energy to help you sleep or watch TV. Listen to your body and don't let your taste buds take over your brain. Have a nice tall glass of water!

This simply gives your body a 10-12 hour break to use up what you've got in there.

Many people consume a large number of their calories at night. Your body is shutting down for the night. You do not need as many calories as you did at breakfast. Although you may *feel* like a nighttime snack, your body actually doesn't need it.

<u>Want versus Need. The battle is on!</u>
You want it, you know it will taste good. In fact, you can taste it at the tip of your tongue. But the only reason you want it is for those taste buds. A fight with yourself in your head may ensue. Fight the fight. Just say no.

Simply tell yourself, it's not an option.

Not eating past 8:00 pm (for me) was a way to control unnecessary calories going into my body at a lousy time (watching TV and needing a snack, looking in the fridge when I got bored). This was the way I broke myself of a nasty habit. Closing the kitchen closed my calorie consumption.

Doing this and this alone may help you lose a couple pounds this week!

THIS WEEK

FOLLOW YOUR PLAN

PEE CLEAR

WATCH YOUR PORTIONS
*(7 out of 10)

25 GRAMS OF FIBER

CLOSE THE KITCHEN AT 8 PM
*(Start and end with water)

*Tips

- Use your week three MASTER PLAN to help you map out week four.
- Repeat your favorites from the week and try something new.
- Get together or phone a friend! Call each other when it's 9 pm and you want to open you refrigerator. Help convince each other that water is the better option.

YOUR WEEK FOUR WORKSHEET AND GROCERY LIST:

MONDAY

Breakfast:

Snack:

Lunch:

Snack:

Dinner:

TUESDAY

Breakfast:

Snack:

Lunch:

Snack:

Dinner:

WEDNESDAY

Breakfast:

Snack:

Lunch:

Snack:

Dinner:

THURSDAY

Breakfast:

Snack:

Lunch:

Snack:

Dinner:

FRIDAY

Breakfast:

Snack:

Lunch:

Snack:

Dinner:

SATURDAY

Breakfast:

Snack:

Lunch:

Snack:

Dinner:

SUNDAY

Breakfast: Lunch: Dinner:

Snack: Snack:

GROCERY LIST

Fruits and Veggies:

Whole Grains (Cereals, Breads, Rice ect..):

Dairy (Cheese, Eggs, Yogurt, Milk, ect..) :

Dips, Sauces & Spices:

Meats and Fish:

Other :

DAILY PLAN

Breakfast:

Snack:

Lunch:

Snack:

Dinner:

DAILY PLAN

Breakfast:

Snack:

Lunch:

Snack:

Dinner:

DAILY PLAN

Breakfast:

Snack:

Lunch:

Snack:

Dinner:

DAILY PLAN

Breakfast:

Snack:

Lunch:

Snack:

Dinner:

DAILY PLAN

Breakfast:

Snack:

Lunch:

Snack:

Dinner:

DAILY PLAN

Breakfast:

Snack:

Lunch:

Snack:

Dinner:

DAILY PLAN

Breakfast:

Snack:

Lunch:

Snack:

Dinner:

DAILY PLAN

Breakfast:

Snack:

Lunch:

Snack:

Dinner:

Now you've mastered the tips you need to help you live a healthy life style. You're still treating yourself to the things you enjoy, just in moderation! And if you ever forget, here they are again:

<u>Your rules to live by!</u>

LAY OUT YOUR PLAN

PEE CLEAR

WATCH YOUR PORTIONS
(Eat until you're a 7 out of 10)

GETTING 25 GRAMS OF FIBER A DAY

CLOSE THE KITCHEN AT 8 PM
(Start and end with water)

When in doubt, phone a friend!

The Carbohydrate Factor

Can you eat carbohydrates and still lose weight? Yes, you can. But let me stress these two very important points.

1) Make sure you are eating them in moderation and in their correct portion sizes.
2) Make sure you are eating whole grains.

As I mentioned earlier, the main theme in all diet programs is balancing calories that you are eating with those that you are using. Programs tend to cut carbohydrates because:

1) Carbohydrates are simply filler.
2) Many people don't know what a real serving size is and tend to over do it.

The reality is, you will have more success with your weight loss goals if you focus your attention on lean protein and vegetables as your main source of nutrients and enjoy carbohydrates in small portions; for example ¾ of a cup of cooked whole grain pasta.

Protein not only helps keep you feeling full (it takes longer to digest) but it also helps curb unwanted cravings! [35]

Life's Little Curve Balls

Let Your Peeps in on It

Tell the people you love (and who love you) about the journey you are embarking on. I truly believe this is a major key to being successful. You'd be surprised how many people step up to help you achieve your goals. Who knows, you may even inspire someone else to join your team! Telling people will provide a strong network for you to rely on. It will also hold you accountable to someone other than yourself.

There will be people out there who want to sabotage your efforts, maybe not maliciously, but it's still important to look out for them. I call these people frien-emies. I don't know if it's because they are jealous or simply don't like to eat unhealthy food alone, but they are the ones who will say " Split the double chocolate oreo cheesecake with me, I don't want to eat it alone." or "Stay and have one more drink with me, please!" In the back of your head just know that these people feel guilty about what they are eating and think that if they have someone doing it with them, it all of the sudden makes it okay. Don't fall into this trap! Because what happens is this; they are now munching on nachos free of guilt and you are munching on them filled with guilt purely to make your friend feel better. <u>Don't eat for other people, eat for yourself</u> and just say, no thanks!

Going Out to Restaurants

You don't have to avoid restaurants. You obviously don't want to go to a restaurant every day because restaurant food tends to be high in salt and fat no matter how healthy the menu seems. If you have dinner plans with friends, a date with a loved one or simply feel like going out for dinner, put it on your PLAN. Most restaurants these days have menus online. Google the restaurant and have a look at their menu. Decide what you are going to eat <u>before you go</u>. *Know before you go!* A big menu with lots of yummy options can be intimidating and tempting. But if you go in with a PLAN, you'll stick to it. This will stop you from making bad choices at the restaurant. If that breadbasket is not on your PLAN, it ain't going in your mouth!

If you don't have time to find the menu online, or simply can't find it. Here are a few tips to help you at the restaurant:

- Ask the waiter to put half your meal in a take-away container <u>before</u> it comes to the table. If you never saw it, you won't miss it.
- If you're having pasta, have it in a marinara sauce, and be sure to use the first tip.
- Look for grilled, baked or broiled options.
- If you're desperate for the breadbasket, limit yourself to one piece.

- Side salad with dressing on the side goes a long way!
- Switch up your sides from starchy, heavy ones to steamed or grilled veggies.
- Have a glass of wine and enjoy it. Sip it slowly. Have just one glass.
- Avoid buffets.

Fast Food

It's amazing what you can find on the Internet these days. All your favorite restaurants have nutritional information online. If you are someone that tends to frequent fast food restaurants, for example, you can still go, but just watch what you order. Be it McDonald's, Wendy's, Subway or Taco Bell, all you need to know about their menu will be online. *Know before you go*! Many of the chains now have "healthier" options. Decide what you can have as well as its serving size (the smaller the better). Having a PLAN will help you stick to it.

I love "In and Out Burger." Love it. When we pull into the drive through, I have two protein burgers (lettuce instead of a bun) without special sauce and a couple of my husband's fries. I've gotten my fast food fix, without ruining my PLAN!

- A great idea at <u>most</u> fast food chains would be to have a kids' meal. (Try to get nutritional information if you can, because some kids' meals may seem small but you'd be surprised what's in 'em).
- Remember, we're eating till we're a 7 out of 10 on a hunger scale and using water to help fill us up.

Donuts at the Office

You get to the office and "Joe" or "Susie" has brought in a dozen donuts. I'm sure they look delicious, I'll give you that. But let me ask you this, when you woke up this morning did you crave a donut? Probably not. And if you did desperately want one, I would have told you to stop at the store and pick a small one up. But, now that it's in front of you at work, you want it, but not because you actually wanted it an hour ago. An hour ago, it didn't exist. In situations like these, I have a general rule. I won't eat something just because it's there. I have to have wanted it before it got there. Just because someone puts it in front of me does not all of a sudden give me permission to eat it.

I know it's so easy to say, *"Oh, I didn't want this before so I shouldn't eat it now!"* Believe me, I know you will spend at least an hour or so throughout the day thinking about the goodness in the office kitchen and explaining to yourself why you should or should not eat it. You'll even probably walk by it on purpose to play mean tricks with yourself. Staying healthy is as much a mind game as anything. You have to be able to say no to yourself and actually listen. It's tough but it's 100% doable!

Instead, try making a cup of coffee or tea. These brews tend to tame the taste-buds. Throw a stick of minty gum in your mouth, but stay away from sweet flavors like watermelon or strawberry because the sweet taste will just activate those taste buds you are trying to quell and make it harder. And for goodness' sake, stay away from the kitchen! I'm not saying don't have a treat! I am saying have a treat on <u>your terms</u>. When you really, really want it, and in moderation of course!

Booze

I would recommend you only have one glass, no more than twice a week. If you can go without it, I would <u>highly recommend it</u>. I'm not trying to rob you of your enjoyment; just know that if you are choosing to drink alcohol:

More than one glass may SLOW your metabolism down!

- Alcohol dehydrates you. As we learned in the water section, your metabolism needs water to function properly. [30]

- Alcohol depresses the central nervous system, making your metabolism less efficient. (Less fat will be burned off and more will be stored!) [31]

- Alcohol is a carbohydrate. You're basically drinking sugar water, yet another thing that will cause your body to store instead of burn. [32]

Keep that metabolism *metabulous*!!

Friends for Dinner

If you are going to friends for dinner, ask what you can bring along to help. Maybe you can contribute to the meal in a healthful way. Find out what's on the menu. You have secretly coaxed your friend into telling you what she's making and now you have a PLAN. And remember, whatever you make, make it healthy! If you can swing it, *know before you go!* Going in with an idea of what's on the menu and how much you can eat will help you to not over indulge with company.

The important thing is not to feel like you have to say no to anything. Just try to remember what your portion sizes look like and <u>eat in moderation</u>. Remember, 7 out of 10.

For example, let's say your friend is making lasagna! Delicious! PLAN for it. Have one small slice and don't go back for seconds. Fill up on salad. Be proud of yourself for not having that second piece and for skipping the wine (or only having half your glass), and for goodness' sake, enjoy that delicious lasagna.

Entertaining

This one is easy! You're planning the meal so you know what you're making! *Know* your portions before the guests arrive. Serve yourself once. Have the two appetizers that are on your PLAN and the half-serving of cake you wrote down for the night. Just stick to your PLAN.

Kids' Birthday Parties

This can be tough. Lots of goodies, and if you have a sweet tooth like me, it's a challenge. What do I do? I pick a treat. One treat. At the end of the party, I have my treat. (I save it for the end as to have less possibility of struggling to go for seconds.) If pizza is the only thing served, I have a slice. And I don't feel bad about it because one slice of pizza is just fine. It's the pizza (times three or four) and chips and soda and, and, and…that is the problem.

Taunting Leftovers

Unhealthy leftovers, from potato chips to cake to pizza and even stuffing, get tossed in the garbage! Without guilt. Better in the garbage than on my thighs, thank you very much! I am never shy to throw my unhealthy leftovers out, no matter what the event. And when I'm at a friend's house and they offer me a "care package" of left over desserts, I politely say thank you, but no.

Hide–and-Go-Eaters

I know you're out there and you're not alone. You would be surprised at the number of people who sneak food. This is the worst type of eating because it's with extreme guilt. Not only do you wolf your food down without a chance to even enjoy it, but the guilt you experience after is awful! It's a beat-myself free-for-all! Why torture yourself? If you're embarrassed to eat something in front of someone for fear of what they may think, chances are you shouldn't be eating it. And the truth is, whether you're eating McDonald's in your car or grabbing a chocolate bar from your secret stash, just because no one sees you eat it doesn't mean it doesn't count. You are accountable for your actions. The burger and fries you ate in hiding is still over 1000 calories even if you're the only one who knows you ate it.

You're Eating Healthy and Your Significant Other is Not

You're munching on salad and your husband is slurping cream sauce covered noodles. This can be really tough. My suggestion is not always realistic for every relationship but I'll give it to you.

The PLAN should not affect your everyday life. In fact, it will make meal times easier as you will have family dinners already PLANNED out. No last-minute calls for take-out or struggles to put a meal together.

On the occasions that involve ordering in and eating out, ask your partner to try to avoid your weaknesses with you. Going at it as a team makes it so much easier. But not everyone is up for the challenge and if your loved one is not game, never fear, here are some helpful suggestions:

You love pizza and know that one slice is just not possible yet. Your loved one "feels" like pizza. Very nicely make an alternate suggestion, hopefully they can hold off on the pizza until you are not around to watch it. Maybe they will have pizza at the office for lunch tomorrow.

Another example: You love Italian. PLAN your meal before you go. Skip the bread, as Italian tends to have enough carbohydrates. Whatever you decide to order, half it before it comes to the table. I like to half things before they come so I have the satisfaction of finishing my meal. I find that if I simply tell myself I will only eat half of what comes, by the time the waiter rolls around to pick up my plate I've lost all will power and my plate is empty.

If you feel you don't have the strength just yet, find out what your loved one would order and make a healthy version at home. It's so easy to find healthy recipes of your favorites online.

Staying Clear of Danger!

Sometimes it's just not worth it to test yourself. Try not to keep things in the house that you know you just cannot eat in proper portions. Don't put them on your PLAN if you don't think you can swing them in moderation just yet. As you get better with portions, you can begin to try to put old favorites on your PLAN and test your moderation skills. These skills take work and time. I still work on mine everyday!

Do things like:
* <u>Pack a lunch</u> for a Saturday out with the family.
* <u>Pack snacks</u> when you're going someplace where they do something mean like pop fresh Caramel Kettle Corn. Ugh! The smell is a conspiracy, I swear!
* <u>PLAN ahead</u> whenever you can! I always have a one-ounce package of nuts in the car.

<u>***Being prepared is key!**</u>
If you're hungry you will reach for the quickest thing. If it happens to be the cut-up veggies or the apple you brought with you, you're golden!*

Worst-Case Scenario

I like to ask myself the worst-case scenario question. What is the worst thing that will happen if I don't have the basket of bread? Will I enjoy dinner any less? What is the worst thing that will happen if I stay away from the potato salad with mayo at the party? Will I have a horrible time? What is the worst thing that will happen if I have one glass of wine and stop at that? What is the worst thing that will happen if I don't go back for seconds? Because really, in truth, there are no horrible consequences to any of these, and in fact there are wonderful benefits. Sure, you may be uncomfortable. You may spend 10 minutes talking yourself down from the breadbasket in your head. But know this: the more you say *no* the easier it gets. I promise.

If You Jump Ship

Remember, treat yourself as if you would your best friend. Would you scream at your best friend for having two cupcakes. No. In fact, if you do overindulge, *enjoy it.* Never, I mean never, eat with guilt. You have to enjoy what you decided to eat. <u>Eating is a conscious decision</u>. It's not a punishment to have a slice of cake, it's a treat, so "treat" it as such. Don't beat yourself up.

What you should not do is throw caution to the wind and start to eat everything in sight because "you messed up, you might as well go for it!" If you had a flat tire would you pull over to the side of the road and slash all your other tires or would you simply call for help? Have your treat, and stop at that. But remember, if you do over-indulge, this is life. We are all human. Just make sure to stop yourself when you get your brain back and make the next thing that goes into your mouth healthy and size-appropriate. Don't wait till the next day or Monday to do it.

Life is full of ups and downs, twists and turns. Changing the way you eat will be as well. Expect it. Embrace it.

Don't give up on yourself because you had one bad meal, a bad day, a bad weekend or even a bad week. This does not mean you've "come off" THE PLAN. It's now how you live! Just come back to it. Remember, everyday is a new day. It doesn't matter what yesterday was, it's today!

Look, no one is 100% perfect with their diet 100% of the time. You should not abandon ship because you think you messed up. You have to stick with it. If you are good 80% of the time, you are still going to see huge changes. If you do indulge and have three slices of pizza, it's probably better than the six you would have had before reading this book. It may take a bit longer to see results, but you will still see the results. This is by no means a free ticket to over-eating. This is merely me, reminding you that you're human, not superhuman. We all trip up, but we get back on that ship and keep sailing ahead, never backwards.

Impulse Buys

We've all done it. We see that bag of Doritos, or that box of chocolate covered almonds and think, "Oh, if I buy this now (I mean, it is on sale) I'll just keep it in the cupboard for later." The reality is, if you buy it, you're going to eat it. You're not buying treats for them to sit on your shelf at home. If it's not something you really, really, really want right now, don't buy it. When you do want those Doritos, make a special trip and get a small bag. If it's just sitting in the house, you'll eat it just because it's there.

What About My Favorite Snacks?

A very dear friend asked me, "Well, what if I want Triscuits and hummus as a snack? Can I have that?" Yes. Have it! Read the ingredients on the box! If you're okay with what's in there, have a look at the serving size. Pull out your eight crackers and spoon out your serving of hummus and enjoy! This applies to whatever you choose for your meals and snacks. Read the labels, follow the serving sizes.

Testing Your Night Time Cravings

It's 10pm. You're hungry, or so you think. I bet you could really go for that frozen yogurt in the freezer. (It is yogurt after all!) Or maybe just finish off that bag of chips in the cupboard (there's really only crumbs left!) Now, are you *really* hungry or are you just bored and noshey. Here is a great test! Ask yourself this: Would I eat a chicken breast or a hard boiled egg right now? Your answer, probably not.

If you did answer no, then grab a tall glass of water and occupy yourself. You may need to talk yourself down from the ice cream or chips, but let your mind win – not your tummy. If you did answer yes, then by all means, boil yourself an egg and eat it! Maybe you didn't eat enough at dinner.

What Are You Craving?

Sometimes when we think we're craving something, we're actually not. We may just be tired, lonely, anxious, upset, irritated, or even bored. At these times, sometimes it can feel like things will just be better if you eat. Because of these misleading pangs, one must always try figure out what you're really 'craving' before you step into the kitchen. Easier said than done, I know. But here's what you can try to do. Before you reach for that night time treat, ask yourself: What am I actually craving? Have I eaten enough today? Or is it even food? Am I really just feeling tired and irritable? Maybe I need to sleep. I'm going to bed! Am I feeling kind of lonely right now? Instead of over-eating, call a friend! Often we just want to busy ourselves, and eating is an easy way to "feel" busy. It can be used as an easy distraction (a way of changing your internal channel) from what your body, mind and soul truly needs. Next time, try to ask yourself what you're really craving!

Rewarding Yourself

Treat yourself. Reward yourself. But please, <u>not with food</u>.

Set little goals for yourself. When you reach 'em, buy yourself something pretty!
Get your nails done.
Go to the movies.
Hit the links at your favorite course.
Whatever it is, enjoy it!

One of my clients gave herself $10 for every pounds she lost. When she steped on the scale after a month and saw 9 pounds, she had $90 to spend at her favorite store!

Why Can't I Reward Myself With Food?

First of all, it's called cheating, not rewarding.

* For most a cheat day is a free-for-all eating feast that starts at dawn and goes till dusk. But on the PLAN, you can have everything you want, simply in moderation. There should be no reason or need to "cheat" and go on an eating bender.

* No recovering alcoholic gets a day to drink his/her face off. Booze is simply off-limits. Foods that trigger overeating should be off-limits too. Know your weaknesses. Superman has Kryptonite. I have cinnamon rolls! I know what I have to stay away from. No kidding. Someone walks into a room with your Kryptonite, fly away, Supes! Because the only thing worse than seeing and smelling cinnamon rolls is watching other people eating cinnamon rolls.

* Just because you were really good for six days does not mean you "deserve" a day off. Those days were spent working hard to form new habits and trying to maintain a calorie deficit. Remember, 3500 calories is a pound. In one (yes, one) cheat day you can eat enough calories to make all your work from the past six days disappear! You have no idea how easy it is to consume 3500 calories. But I think you know how hard it is to burn it off.

* Cheat days will also throw you off- balance. The day after a cheat, you will have all these delicious salty and sweet tastes at the tip of your tongue. It's now that much harder to make the right choices and stick to them.

* *Did you know?* Studies suggest it takes two to four weeks to form a habit.

My personal opinion? 21 days. Three weeks. If you stick to your healthy eating for 12 days and then go loco on day 13, you may have put yourself back at square one. But if you can last for 21 days, you have the power to kick a serious sugar craving habit!

* If you are trying to lose weight, it most probably means you have fat stored up. You need to eat fewer calories than your body needs so that it's forced to draw its energy from your fat stores. Cheating is not going to help at all.

I'm not saying don't have pancakes. I'm saying don't reward yourself with them! Have them because you really, really want them. But, have two instead of six.

Look, whatever it is you really, really want, have it. Measure it, make sure you're having one portion, and enjoy it. There should be no need to cheat.

Weighing In

The following is a list of some of the things that can affect your number on the scale: [33, 34]

* Weight naturally fluctuates daily anywhere from 1 – 5 pounds!

* For women, during a menstrual cycle, you retain water, causing bloating:
  The number on your scale may temporarily rise.

* Sodium rich foods like soy sauce the night before will cause water retention:
  The number on your scale may temporarily rise.

* Drinking alcohol the night before will actually dehydrate you:
  The number on your scale may temporarily shrink.

* If you have had anything to eat or drink before the weigh in:
  The number on your scale may temporarily rise.

How often should you weight yourself?

I strongly suggest you weigh yourself every four to six weeks, first thing in the morning, naked and after your morning pee. Give yourself four or even six weeks to make a dent. Don't pressure yourself with a scale. This is a lifestyle, remember.

Allow your clothes and the way you feel to dictate how great you are doing. Don't let a number on some silly scale tell you if you're doing well or not.

Feel good about yourself because of the actions you are taking, not because a scale said you weighed 1.375 pounds less than you did the Friday before. Why hand over all that power to an inanimate object?

Our minds like to play tricks on us. I have seen this too many times not to say it doesn't happen:

a) People step on that scale daily and see they have lost weight! Woo hoo! They relax a little, having that second helping as a pat on the back. <u>Danger</u>!

b) People step on the scale daily and don't see any results! Or worse, a weight gain! They get bummed out and resort to their good old favorite! Comforting themselves with a bit of love from food. <u>Danger</u>!

Having said all that, I can totally understand wanting to see your progress. I get it. I'm a girl. I'm human. So, if you are going against my better judgment, do not weigh yourself more than once a week and:

* Understand all the things that can affect your weight.
* Make sure you have found ways to reward yourself other than with food.
* Know that if the number doesn't budge, or even climbs, there are many reasons this can happen:

> * You could have just had a bad week.
> * You could have eaten a lot of salt.
> * You could have developed some muscle mass.
>   (Woo hoo! Your metabolism is becoming metabulous!)
> * You could have lost an inch from your waist even though the scale tells you you're up a pound. *(Hooray for muscle!)*

I would like to end on the same note I began on. I designed the PLAN so that you don't have to give up the things you love. Food is social! It is front and center when you get together with friends, family and loved ones. We celebrate with it, holiday with it and sometimes we cry with it! This is why I say if you have a love of wine, have a glass! Enjoy your glass! But stop at that.

What we put in our mouths is conscious. We choose what we eat.
We can choose to ignore it, or we can stop ignoring it and pay attention.

My Favorite Foods

The following is a list of my favorite foods. These foods make my list simply because they are good for me and I eat them a lot! There are many other foods out there that are just as good for you; they have just not found their way into my refrigerator. I always try to have my house stocked with my favorites. The more good stuff I have in the house, the less likely I am to reach for the bad stuff.

Protein
I love having lean protein in my freezer. It's easy to defrost and quick to grill or bake. Lean protein is nutrient rich, low in calories, low in fat and fills you up!

Did you know?
Protein is the most difficult macro nutrient for your body to digest. This means you actually burn more calories digesting protein then you do digesting carbohydrates or fat. And because it takes a bit longer to digest, you stay full longer too. [35]

In my freezer or fridge you will often find:

Boneless skinless chicken breasts	Lean pork chops
Turkey breasts	Lean ground turkey
Tuna	Lean ground chicken
Salmon	White fish
Shrimp	Eggs and egg whites

* I know there is much research about mercury in fish. I am not a doctor. So please consult your physician before eating copious amounts of fish. However, I am a firm believer that there are many benefits to eating fish; again I am not an authority. Anything outside of moderation is likely too much.

Nuts
These are great as a snack. You can add them to a salad or spread them on some toast or even munch on them as is. Just make sure you measure out a one-ounce portion. I sometimes replace butter or oil in a baking recipe with natural nut butter. You get an extra protein boost and a preservative-free ingredient, plus some Omega 3 fatty acids (which are great for your brain and your heart). These are my personal favorites:

Natural peanut butter
Natural almond butter
Natural cashew butter
Pistachios in shell, unsalted

Raw unsalted almonds
Raw unsalted brazil nuts
Raw unsalted cashews
Walnuts, unsalted

Vegetables and Fruit

Any and all fruits and vegetables have great health benefits. Just because they're not on this list, doesn't necessarily mean they're not great. All are high in water and fiber, full of nutrient-rich vitamins, minerals and antioxidants. There is so much variety in fruits and vegetables and so many different flavors and textures. They truly are nature's candy!

Sweet potatoes
Spinach
Broccoli
Asparagus
String beans
Celery
Carrots
Cucumber

Brussels sprouts
Beets
Zucchini
Spaghetti squash
Butter lettuce
Green beans
Sugar snap peas
Kale

Kiwi
Apples
Grapefruit
Strawberries
Raspberries
Mango

Blackberries
Pineapple
Peaches
Bananas
Grapes
Pomegranate

Carbohydrates and Whole Grains

Full of fiber-rich nutrients, carbohydrates are your body's preferred energy source. It's what you use as fuel.[29] A whole grain product rich in fiber will take more time to digest, keeping you full longer (this is a great asset for weight loss).

Sprouted grain breads, wraps and English muffins
Whole grains breads
Whole grain wraps
Whole grain pastas

Brown rice
Quinoa
Couscous
Wild rice
Pearl barley

Dairy

Not only is it high in protein and rich in calcium (great for building and maintaining bone density), scientists now believe that dairy actually helps our body process and rid itself of fat. [36]

Low-fat or fat-free milk
Low-fat cottage cheese
Low-fat or fat-free yogurt
2 % milkfat cheese

Beans
Folate, potassium, fiber, antioxidants and protein; all that and still low in fat.

Garbanzo beans	Kidney Beans
Black beans	Lentils

What I look for in a packaged product:
* It must taste good.
* If it's in a box or a bag I try to find it as unprocessed as I can. I don't always succeed but I try. This means I look to see if all the ingredients are ones that I can understand. Real food, not chemicals. Again, the operative word is try.
* I make sure there is no partially hydrogenised oil of any kind (trans fat).
* I try to avoid high fructose corn syrup.
* I look for little to no saturated fat in the product.
* If the product contains any form of sugar, I try to make sure it's closer to the bottom of the ingredients list. (Ingredients are listed in order of how much is in the product, from most to least.)
* There must be something in whatever it is I eat that is good for me.
   For example: A Gnu Bar is great to grab on the go: it's preservative-free, high in fiber and low in fat.

A word of caution: ready-made meals tend to be high in sodium. Based on a 2000 calorie a day diet, the FDA recommends you do not have more than 2400 mg of Sodium in a day. [26] (That is equivalent to approximately 1 teaspoon of salt.)

I'm not perfect. Everything I put into my mouth is not chemical-free, pure as can be, completely free of saturated fats and 100% good for me. I try, and if 80% of the time I'm good, I know it's way better than 30% or even 50%.

Here are a few of my favorite products:

Cereals

Shredded Wheat	Kashi Go Lean
Weetabix	Kashi 7 Grain Puff
Steel Cut Irish Oatmeal	Quinoa Puffs

Bars
Bars are for emergencies only. I take real food over a bar any day.

Gnu Bars	Lara Bars	The Simply Bar

A note about sprouted grain bread
Sprouted grain bread is my bread of choice because it's full of healthy, whole (not refined) ingredients that are high in protein and fiber. "Sprouting" the grains makes them easier for your

body to digest and process the nutrients and vitamins in the grain. Many sprouted grain products even form a complete protein!

Breads
Ezekiel 4:7 Sprouted Grain
Ezekiel Sprouted English Muffins
Ezekiel Sprouted Grain Cinnamon Raisin
Sprouted Bread, Buns, Wraps of any kind

Dairy
0% Liberte Greek Yogurt
Fage Greek Yogurt
Organic Fat-Free Milk
Organic 1% Milk
2 % Milk fat Cheeses

A note about 0% Greek style yogurt
I love this stuff because of its simple ingredients. It's rich and creamy in texture and the amount of protein you get in a serving is astounding!

Treats
Chapman's Vanilla Frozen Yogurt
Vita Muffins
70% Dark Chocolate
Yoga Chips
Yogen Fruz *blended low-fat yogurt with frozen mixed berries*
Natural home made popped popcorn

Into Exercise

Let's make that heart of yours pump!

Here are three different ways to begin working exercise into your daily routine. All are important. Don't try to fit all three in at once. Start with one that works within your lifestyle and go from there. Slowly introduce exercise so that it becomes a habit. Once it's a habit, finding the time will seem much easier.

Why do we have to do this again?

We do it to burn calories, of course! That's probably the primary reason people exercise. You'll feel good about yourself and you'll look great. But exercise is also like little lessons for your heart. The more your heart gets to practice, the better it will become. The less it gets to practice, the more it forgets what it should know.

I know you know all this, but just as a refresher: Your heart is responsible for delivering blood throughout your body. Your blood carries oxygen and nutrients (from the food you eat and the air you breathe) to your muscles and organs to keep them working. When you exercise, your heart is forced to deliver more blood into your body. Your muscles need the extra energy. With exercise, your heart becomes stronger and teaches itself to deliver more blood with every pump; it will even begin to do this when you're not exercising. Your heart will now have to pump fewer times then it used because each pump carries more blood, lowering your blood pressure. [38,39] This will not happen if you stay seated, I promise.

What is the difference between exercise and daily activity?
Whereas with exercise you want to be a bit breathless, daily activity is basically getting off your couch, walking to the store, taking the stairs, going for a leisurely walk. Daily activity is not exercise. But it's just as important.

Did you know ?
Some studies suggest that people who fidget and move about can actually burn an additional 100-300 calories a day. [40]

1. For daily activity as well as exercise, studies suggest healthy individuals should be taking 10,000 steps a day. [41] Sounds like a lot, I know, but once you realize how easy it is to rack up steps, you'll be well on your way. It's important to increase the amount of walking and moving you are doing. I suggest you buy yourself a pedometer. You can get them at any drug store or pharmacy for about 10 dollars. Clip it onto your waist and start moving.

Work your way up to, and then stay at, your 10,000 steps. Make it a game for yourself. Team up with someone and see who can rack up the most steps.

I know these might sound like silly pieces of advice you've heard 100 times, but they're true.

Walk when you can.
Park far away.
Take the stairs.
Walk around your block once a day.

2. Every healthy human being should be able to participate in aerobic <u>exercise</u> for a minimum of 30 minutes three times a week. [37, 39]

While performing aerobic exercise, you should be breathing heavily but still be able to have a very light conversation. You should not be breathless or unable to talk.

This is not so you can look like Arnold; this is so your heart can function the way it was designed to. This is for heart health. And of course let's not forget the calories you will burn.

Work your way up to 30 minutes of aerobic exercise. You can speed walk, jog, bike ride, use the cross trainer or elliptical machine, rock climb, wrestle, trampoline, swim, strength train with circuits—whatever your little heart desires!

Ideally 30 minutes three to five times a week is great. Realistically, I know that 30 minutes can seem like a huge chunk. Many people avoid it all together because they can't seem to find 30 minutes. But I bet they can find 10.

Ten minutes three times a day or 15 minutes twice a day still equals 30 minutes.

You don't have to do it all at once to reap the rewards. Split it up!

And if you only have 10 or 15 minutes one day, it's a lot better than zero.
Always do as much as you can, even if it's not 30 minutes.

Once you reach this goal you can begin to play with intensity and timing, training your heart to function even more effectively and burning even more calories. But that's for another book.

Our bodies are going to be with us for a long time. We have to keep them moving and well-oiled if we expect them to last and work the way we want them to.

This is also why strength training is important. Again, no Arnold here, just health for now and for your future.

3. <u>Why Strength training is important.</u>[42]

* Strengthens your heart while strengthening your muscles.

* Increase the rate at which you metabolize food. The more muscle you have, the harder your body has to work to fuel those muscles. Therefore you will burn more calories, even at rest!

* Aids in bone density, especially important for women.

* Helps with balance, gait and your center of gravity.

* Makes you stronger and less prone to injury.

* Helps to repair and restore injuries.

* Makes you feel strong.

The silliest thing happened to me. I was out for a jog and I whipped out. Fell face (well wrist) first onto the hard pavement. I didn't break, bruise or sprain a thing! Not even my wrist, which braced the fall. With my 5-foot-2 frame, I always thought of myself as fragile, especially with a family history of osteoporosis. I have *always* been afraid to fall. And here I was, getting off my sore butt, dusting myself off and walking. I felt so strong! And I know it's because I made myself strong. I worked hard, and it's paying off. I was so happy to have fallen (ridiculous, I know) and so proud of myself for being able to get off my butt.

We need to build a foundation of muscles so that when we are 35 or 45, 55 or 85, we can screw in light bulbs, open pickle jars, walk up and down stairs when the elevator breaks and continue to be calorie-burning machines.

Exercises

The following are exercises you can do in the privacy of your own home with cheap equipment. All you need are resistance bands and a stability ball.

Resistance bands are sold in a variety of different colors.
Although it should say on the box what level you are purchasing, a general rule of thumb is:

> Yellow—Extra Light
> Green—Light
> Blue—Heavy
> Red—Medium
> Black—Extra Heavy

- The wider you stand on the band, the more resistance you will create.

Stability balls come in different sizes designed for different heights.
Although the packaging should direct you to the appropriate ball for your height, a general rule of thumb is:

4'6" - 5'0"	45 cm (17.7")
5'1" - 5'7"	55 cm (21.6")
5'8" - 6'1"	65 cm (25.5")
6'2" - 6'7"	75 cm (29.5")
6'7-$_{1/4}$" and up	85 cm (33.5")

- With all these exercises, please remember to keep a neutral spine. Keep your shoulders down, your feet in line with your hips, your knees over your second and third toes. Keep your core activated in order to prevent your lower back from arching.

Activating your Core
How do you activate your core?

Stand doing nothing. Place your thumb in your belly button and lay your palm flat on your tummy. Notice your fingers are resting near your lower abdomen. From the tips of your fingers, pull in and up using your deep stomach muscles. This is how you properly activate your core. You want to keep your core activated for all weight-bearing exercises. It will protect your lower back, help strengthen your ability to balance as well as build strong stabilizing muscles.

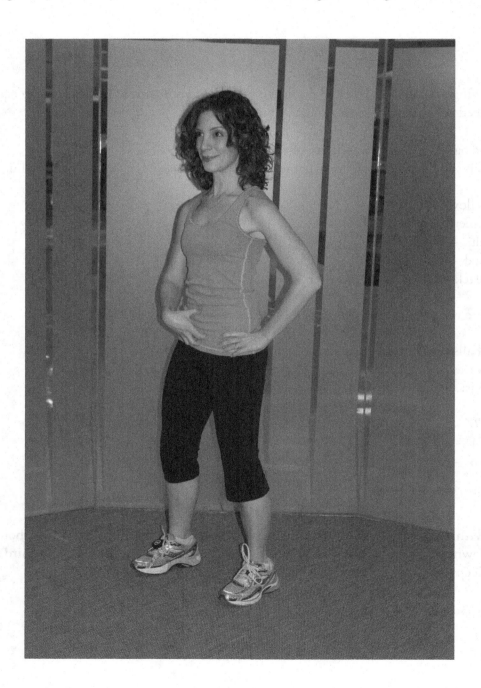

ARMS

a) **Bicep Curls**

Stand with your feet shoulder-width apart, with one or both feet on your exercise band. Keep your shoulders down. Place your arms at your sides. Bend at your elbows, bringing your hands below 90 degrees with your palms facing the ceiling. From here bring the handles to your shoulders and back down. Repeat for 15 repetitions. Be sure to keep your shoulders from rising up and keep those elbows glued to the sides of your body.

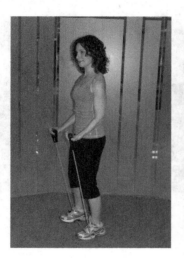 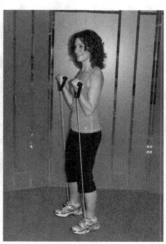

b) **Bicep Hammer Curls**

This is identical to a regular bicep curl except the placement of your hands is a bit different. This time hold the band just below the handles. Bend at your elbows, bringing your hands below 90 degrees. Your palms will be making fists and facing each other in a "hammer" position. From here bring your hands to your shoulders and back down to 90. Repeat 15 times. Once again, your elbows will stay glued to your sides.

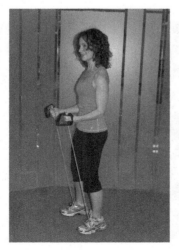 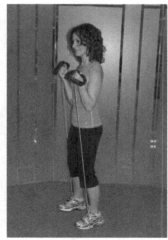

c) **8, 8, 8 Bicep Curl**

You can perform this exercise either as a regular bicep curl or a hammer curl. Begin the exercise with eight repetitions of curls from your original starting position but only curl up to 90-degrees. Follow with eight repetitions of curls from the 90-degree bend at your elbows to the top of the motion at your shoulders. Finish with eight repetitions of a full motion curl.

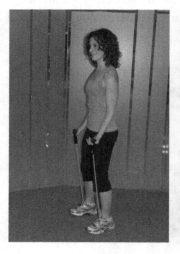 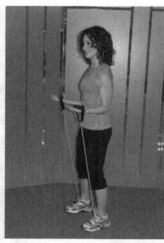 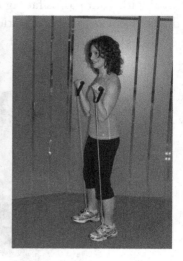

a) **Dips**

Find a very stable chair or bench and crouch down in front of it. Place your palms on the seat so that your fingers hang over the ledge. Lower your body down so that your buttocks move toward the floor, try to stay as close to the bench as possible to protect your shoulders. Come back up to your starting position using your triceps muscles. Work your way up to 15 repetitions.

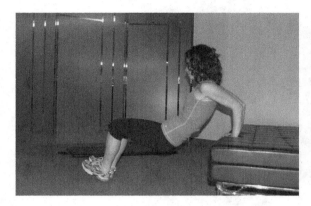 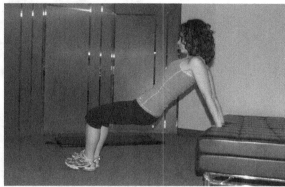

b) **Pull Downs**

Loop your resistance band over a doorway. With your arms at your side, and your elbows in, pull the band toward the floor. When you reach the end of the motion, flare your hands approximately 30 degrees away from your body and then return your hands to a 90-degree bend at your elbows, not higher. Remember to keep those elbows glued to your sides. Repeat 15 times.

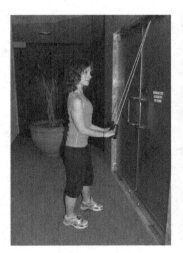 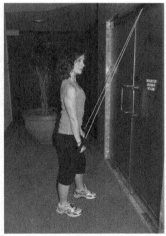

c) **Reverse Triceps Extensions:**

Loop your resistance band over a doorway. Facing away from the door, bend at your hips and bring your elbows in to hug your ears. Keeping your elbows here, push the band away from you and come back to starting. Repeat 15 times.

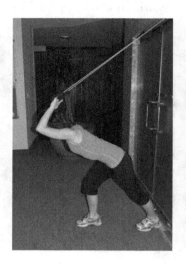 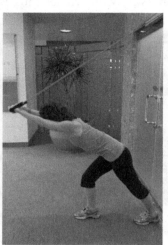

UPPER BODY

a) **Pushups**
Lie facing the floor. Place your hands a bit wider than shoulder distance apart. Keep your core activated to protect your lower back throughout this exercise.

Either:

A) Lift yourself up onto your toes and your hands. Make sure to form a straight line from your heels to your head. You do not want your lower back to sag or your buttocks to rise.

B) Lift yourself up onto your knees and your hands. Make sure to form a straight line from your buttocks to your head. You do not want your lower back to sag or your buttocks to rise.

In both instances, make sure the weight of your body is being pushed through your chest. Push up so that you have full extension in your arms, and then bring yourself as close to the ground as you can without touching. Repeat as many times as you can. Work your way up to 10, then 20, then 30.

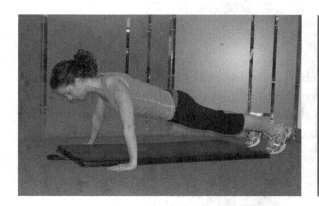
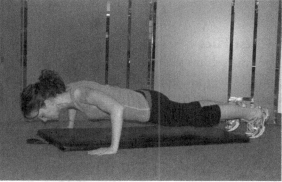
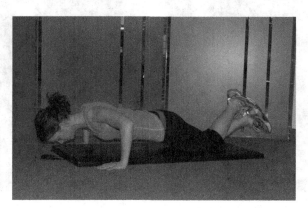

b) **Chest Press**

Loop your resistance band in the jamb of a door with the door hook provided. Stand far enough away from the door so that you create the right amount of resistance for you. Raise your elbows up to shoulder height, keeping your hands in front and in line with your elbows, palms facing toward the ground. Keep your shoulders down and push with your resistance band until your hands meet in front of you. Bring the handles back so that your elbows are in line with your back. 15 repetitions.

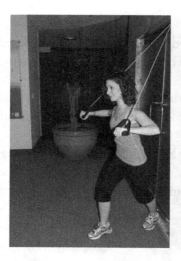 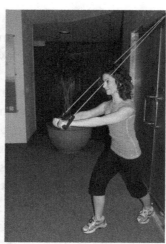

c) **Chest Flies**

Line yourself up the same way you did with the chest press. Instead of having your palms face the ground, they are going to face each other, allowing your elbows to point out. It's as if you were wrapping your hands around a barrel. Push so that your hands meet in front of you and then bring the handles back, allowing your elbows to come in line with your back. Repeat 15 times.

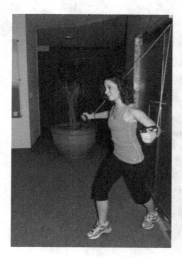 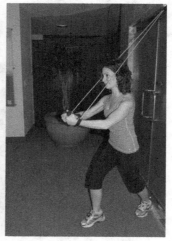

a) Shoulder Raises To Front & Side

Front: In a neutral position with your core activated, stand on your resistance band and hold onto the handles. Keep you shoulders down. Raise your hands in front of you keeping a very slight bend in the elbow and then come back to your starting position. Repeat 15 times.

Side: In a neutral position with your core activated, stand on your resistance band and hold onto the handles. Keep you shoulders down. Raise your hands to your sides (as if you were making a T). Come back to your starting position. Repeat 15 times with each arm.

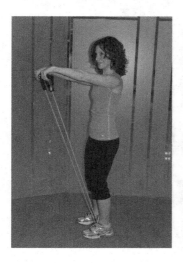 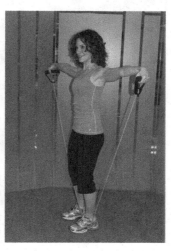

b) Upright Rows

In a neutral position with your core activated, stand on your resistance band, holding the handles. With the handles in front of you and touching each other, raise your hands just below your chin so that your elbows poke out. Bring your hands back down and repeat 15 times. *Remember to keep your shoulders down. They'll want to sneak up!

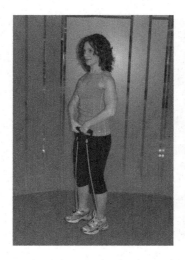 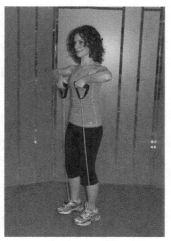

c) **Shoulder Press**

Stand on your exercise band in neutral. Holding onto the handles, form the bottom half of a box with your arms above your head. Your elbows will be bent to 90 degrees and in line with your shoulders. From here, move your arms up toward the ceiling and allow them to meet above your head. Come back to your starting "box" position. 15 repetitions.

* It is important to keep your shoulders from elevating.

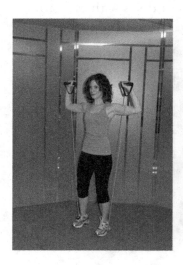 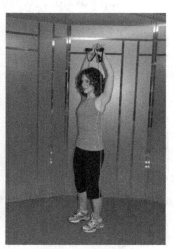

a) **Prone Lateral Raise**

Lie face down on the floor. Bring your arms in front of you to form a Y, thumbs pointing toward the ceiling. In a very small motion, lift your arms, head, and chest off the floor, keeping your head and neck in line with your spine (make sure your chin does not jut out). Bring yourself back to your original position and repeat 15 times.

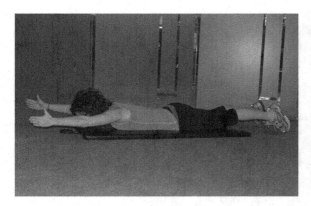 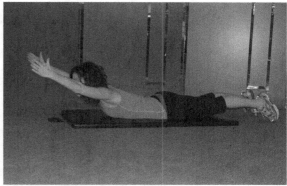

b) **Bent Over Row**

Place your resistance band underneath your feet and hold each handle. Bend over at your hips so that your back is flat. Begin by squeezing your shoulder blades together as if you had a pencil in between them, pull the handles up beside your chest trying to keep your elbows inline with your shoulders. Bring the handles back to your starting position by releasing your shoulder blades and repeat 15 times.

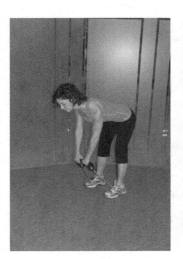 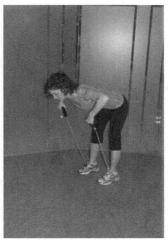

c) **Partial Good Mornings**

Stand in neutral. Cross your hands in front of your body in a mummy position. Allow for a very slight bend in your knees. Bend over at the hips, only as far as you can maintain a flat back, and then with a flat back, come back to your starting position. Keep your core activated and use it to bring yourself back up. *As soon as you feel your back begin to arch, return to neutral. Repeat this exercise 15 times.

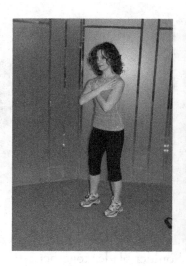 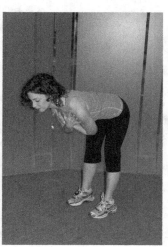

CORE & YOUR CENTER OF GRAVITY

a) **Plank**

Lie face down on the floor. Lift your body onto the tips of your toes and your forearms. Stay here. Try not to let your feet and forearms take over the work. They are merely contact points with the ground. What's holding you up are those muscles deep in your stomach, so you'll need to focus on activating your core. Start holding this position for five or 10 seconds, repeating the exercise up to 10 times. Work your way up to holding for 60 seconds, repeating the exercise two or three times. Activating your core will also help you keep your back flat. Don't let your lower back sag or your butt lift.

* You may also perform this exercise on your knees and work your way up to using your toes.

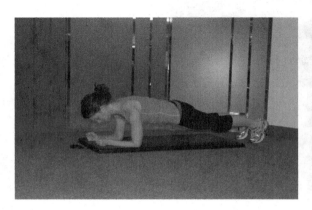 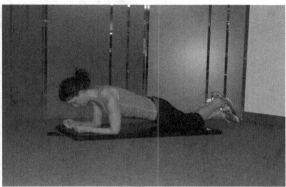

b) **Stability Ball Roll out**

On your knees, punch the lower half of a stability ball. Allow the ball to roll out in front of you until you feel your core stabilizers holding the ball in place. With your core, bring the ball back towards you and repeat.

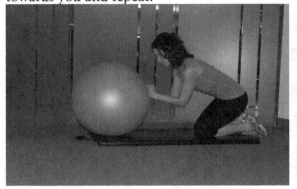 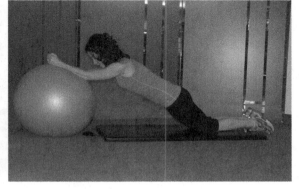

c) Crunch

Lie on your back with your knees bent. Lift your head and shoulders slightly off the ground, activate your core. (You can rest your hands behind your head to support your neck, but don't use your hands to lift your head. Merely rest them there.) When you begin the "crunch" motion, imagine that your ribs are slicing your belly button in half. It is s a very small motion, only 1-2 inches. Hold for two counts and come back to your starting *activated* position. Try never to dip below activation. Work your way up to 25! When you're there, add another set!

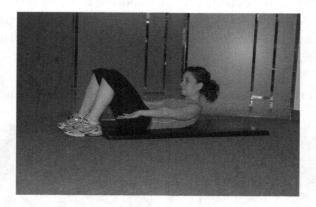

a) Single Leg Point

Stand in a neutral position, feet hip distance apart, knees over your second and third toe. Lift one foot off the ground. Point your foot forward and bring it back (keeping it off the ground). Take your time! Do this on a count of two. One, two, forward. One, two, back. Repeat 10 times. With your foot still in the air, point your foot to the side of your body. One, two side, One two back. Finish on one leg and move to the next.

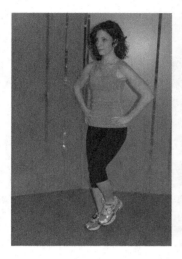 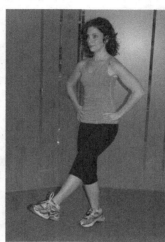 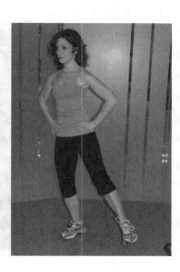

b) Total Body Balance

Stand in a neutral position holding a weight in your hands. (You can use a soup can or water bottle if you don't have any weights.) With the weight in your hands, bring your hands over your head and your foot behind you (on a count of two). Return to your starting position (on a count of two). Repeat 10 times on each leg.

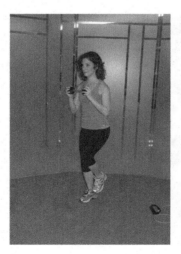 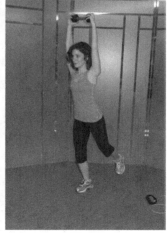

c) Single Leg RDL

Stand in a neutral position. Lift one foot off the ground. Keeping your <u>back straight throughout this movement</u>, bend over at your hips and aim your fingers to touch the floor (go as far as you can while maintaining a flat back). As you lean forward, let your free leg move behind you to help you balance. Repeat 10 times on each leg.

* Keep a slight bend in the knee of the leg you are standing on.

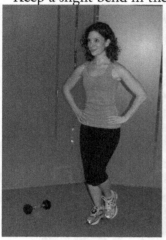 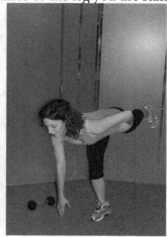

LOWER BODY

a) **Military Squat**

Stand in neutral, feet hip distance apart, knees over your second and third toes. Squat down to 90 degrees. Come back to standing by pushing through your heels and squeezing your buttocks. Activate your core throughout this motion to prevent your lower back from arching. *Try putting a chair behind you and pretending you are going to take a seat. This will help keep your weight behind you to avoid putting unnecessary pressure onto your knees.

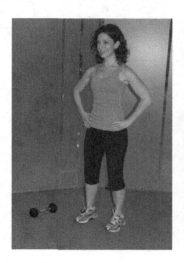 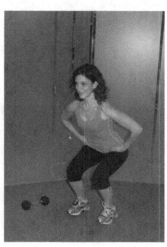

b) **Bridge**

Lie on the floor facing the ceiling. Activate your buttocks by squeezing them as tight as you can and lift them off the floor. Raise your buttocks as high as you can to meet your hips, pushing through your heels. <u>Hold</u> here for three seconds, squeezing your butt the whole time; come back down, about an inch from the ground (still holding the squeeze), but don't let that butt touch the floor. Repeat 15 times. *Watch that your knees don't splay open.

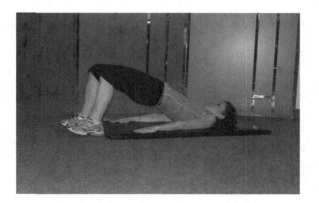

c) **Split Lunge**

Stand in neutral. Step forward with one leg and bend your front knee, feet pointing straight ahead. Allow your back knee to dip so that it almost touches the ground. Keeping your weight in your front heel and back toe, push up to your starting position. Repeat 15 times on each leg. *As your back knee dips toward the ground, you should come straight down without leaning forward; this avoids putting unnecessary pressure on your front knee.

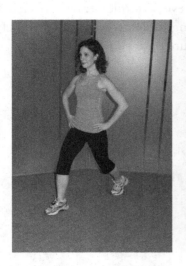
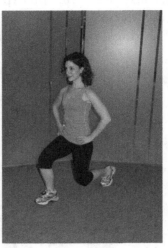

a) Squat and Hold

With your back up against a wall and your feet five or six inches in front of you, bend down to 90 degrees. Push your weight through your heels. Begin by holding here for five seconds and repeat the exercise 10 times. Work your way up to holding 10 seconds, then 20, then 60! (If you can squat and hold for 60 seconds, repeat the exercise two or three times.)

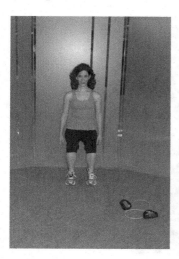

b) Leg Raises With a Hold

Have a seat on a chair. Lift and straighten one leg so that it is level with your chair seat. Keeping your foot flexed, hold here for 10 or 15 seconds, bring your leg back down to your starting position and repeat the exercise 10 times with each leg. You can work your way up to holding this position for one minute!

* Watch that you don't hyperextend your knee!

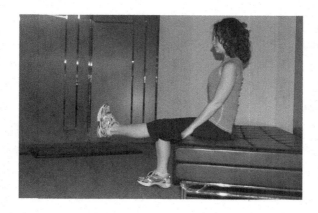

c) Step Up

Find a *very stable* bench or chair. You want your knee to be at about 90 degrees when you step up onto it. Step up onto the chair/bench with your right leg (pushing through your heel) and step down with your left. Step back up with your right and repeat. Finish 10 repetitions on one leg. Repeat with the other leg.

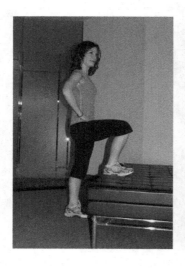 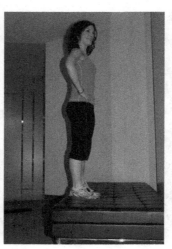

a) Hip Raises

Lie on the floor facing the ceiling. Bend one leg so that your heel is as close to your buttocks as possible, keeping your other leg straight. You essentially want to lift your buttocks off the floor by pushing your weight through the heel of your bent leg. Your straight leg will rise off the floor. Lift your buttocks as high as you can pushing through your heel. Then bring your buttocks back down an inch above the floor. Repeat the motion 15 times on each leg.

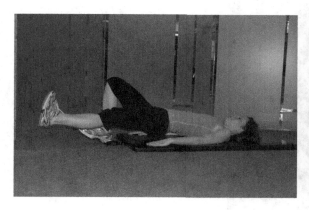 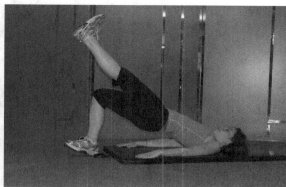

b) Stability Ball Leg Curl

Lie on the floor facing the ceiling. Place both feet on the ball and make sure your toes are pointed toward the ceiling. Lift your buttocks in the air as high as you can. You'll want to focus on keeping your butt lifted for the entire motion of the exercise. Roll the ball toward your butt and then roll it back to your starting position. You'll find that activating your core is very helpful as it will help keep the ball stable and in line. Try performing 12-15 repetitions of this exercise.

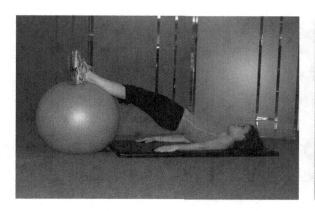 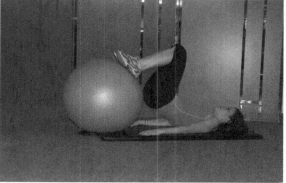

a) **Calf Raise**

Feel free to use the wall for balance. Lift up onto your tippy toes, as high as you can go. Hold for two counts. Bring your heels back down, but do not let them touch the ground. Repeat the movement 20 times slow and 10 times fast.

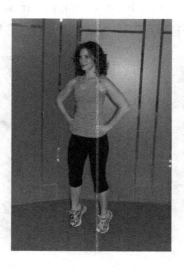

Putting it all together in an easy workout plan!

The following are examples of how I put six exercises together. This will help you get started. Once you have the hang of it, you can go through the list of exercises and pick your own favorites.

These circuits should take no more than 20 minutes. What's 20 minutes two or three times a week? You can even do them in front of the TV.

They are designed to keep you moving, burning the maximum number of calories while you workout.

PLAN 1:
Pick six exercises, one from each muscle group. Perform each exercise 15 times unless otherwise noted and then move to the next without a break. When you have finished your six exercises, take a 60-90 second break.
Repeat this sequence two more times.

Examples:
20 minutes, three days a week (start twice a week and work your way to three times)

Workout 1	Workout 2	Workout 3
8, 8, 8 Bicep Curls	Plank 3 x 20 seconds	Pushups
Military Squat	Bent Over Row	Shoulder Raises -Front & Side
Triceps Pull Down	Bridge	Prone Lateral Raise
Chest Flies	Shoulder Press	Step Up
Leg Raises	S. Ball Hamstring Curl	S. Ball Roll Out
Upright Rows	T. Body Balance x 10 (R & L)	Hammer Curl
60-Second Break	60-Second Rest	60-Second Rest
Repeat 2 more time	Repeat 2 more times	Repeat 2 more time

PLAN 2:
20 minutes, three days a week (start twice a week and work your way to three times)

Upper Body - Day 1	Lower Body - Day 2	Total Body - Day 3
Bicep Curls	Leg Raises	Plank 3 x 20 second hold
Pushups	Total Body Balance	Step Up
Triceps Dips	Hip Raises	Upright Row
Good Mornings	Bridge	Crunch x 20 2 second hold
S. Ball Roll Out	Calf Raises	S. Leg RDL
Shoulder Press	Squat and Hold 5 sec hold x 12	Chest Press
Take a 60-second Break	Take a 60-Second Break	Take a 60-Second Break
Repeat 2 more times	Repeat 2 more times	Repeat 2 more times

Fast Food ? Think Again!

7:30am: You wake up, stumble to the bathroom, brush teeth, shower, get dressed, make-up.

8:00: Make/eat a healthy breakfast.

8:30: You're on the road to work. (So far, so good)

9-Noon: You work your tail off, I'll give you the benefit of the doubt on that. (Here's where it gets interesting.)

12:30- Lunch: You're starving because you didn't have time to grab a snack and you didn't pack one. Gotta find something to eat so you can make your meeting in an hour!

12:45: Arrive at food court (after elevator traffic). Start looking for something to eat, fast.

12:50: Wait in the line of people at Hoagie Heaven (insert your local snack shack here), place your order and wait for them to make it.

1:00: Finally sitting down to eat. Make that *"wolfing down"* because you have to get back to check emails before your meeting at 1:30.

Sound familiar? Good thing you went for fast food...

Not!

If you add up the time it takes to get *to and from* the food court, coupled with the wait times at the counter as you pay and the wait for your food, those minutes fritter away fast. And that's not even including the walk (make that waddle) back to your desk afterwards.

We eat fast food to save time, to make our lives easier (or so we tell ourselves). But the truth is that it always ends up taking 30-40 minutes just to grab a "quick" bite!

Why no avoid this situation all together by checking in with your MASTER PLAN and making yourself a lunch and packing a couple of snacks!

Some of you may say "Whatever, I can grab food and be back at my desk in 20!" I'm not here to argue numbers (well, maybe I am), but if you took a few extra minutes the night before to throw together a lunch and toss in morning/afternoon snacks, you'd actually save more time!

In the end, fast food is not fast at all. The name is actually *misleading*. It's *slow food* because it slows you down time-wise, energy-wise, and even money-wise. Yes, you waste money! You have to work to pay for it. And you know the old adage, time is money.

"C'mon," you say, "fast food is cheap!" Really? If you go to lunch 3-4 days a week, and spend 5-7 dollars for lunch (which is a little low once you include taxes and soda) you're spending over a $1000 a year! That's the price of a vacation!!!! Plus, if you stir up the discipline to bring your lunch and pack some snacks, you'll give yourself a few extra minutes to step away from the rat race (reading, people-watching, listening to music, meditating- and by 'meditating' I mean flipping through trash mags) and cut down on stress.

So why would you work harder and longer to pay for your fast food- sorry *"slow food"*- when you could really just squeeze 5-10 minutes at night and give yourself more time during the day to do something good for yourself?

Want to eat fast food?
<u>Make it yourself.</u>

Thank you to my husband for contributing "Fast Food, Think again"

Recipes and Meal Ideas

Healthy eating ideas for a fast breakfast

Breakfast recipes

Snack ideas

My favorite meal—pizza!

Ideas for packing a lunch

Sandwiches

Chicken & turkey

Stir fry recipes

Ground turkey

Pasta & noodles

Pork chops

Fish & seafood

Salads & dressings

Soups & side dishes

Dessert recipes and quick sweet tooth fix ideas

*Please consider nutritional information as estimates. It is not guaranteed to be 100% accurate.

Healthy eating ideas for a fast breakfast

If you're stuck for breakfast, here are some great ideas:

*Scramble 1 egg and 2 whites, a piece of grain toast and some Canadian back bacon.

*Scramble 1 egg and 2 whites; serve them with a whole grain wrap with salsa, avocado, light cheddar cheese and black beans.

*Make yourself an egg sandwich with a whole grain English muffin, scrambled 1 egg and 2 whites, lettuce, tomato and light cheese or a slice of Canadian bacon.

*Sunnyside up style with a piece of whole grain to dip! Remember eggs and soldiers from when you were a kid!?

*Whole grain cereal and non-fat milk. Top it off with some fresh fruit!

*Whole or sprouted grain toast with peanut butter. Try it open-faced with a sliced banana on top!

* Low-fat cottage cheese with fresh berries.

* Fresh fruit plate (Try: ½ grapefruit, 1 kiwi, sliced pineapple and some berries)

Breakfast Recipes

Oatmeal with Warm Banana

Strawberry Banana Breakfast Bonanza

No Toast French Toast

Cinnamon French Toast

Popeye Pancakes

Salsa Omelet

Goat Cheese Omelet

Egg White & Feta Quesadilla

Bacon, Swiss and Asparagus Frittata

Vegetable and Cheese Crust-less Quiche

Eggs Jenny

Peanut Butter Banana Chocolate Breakfast Cookies

Apple Cinnamon Bombs

5 Banana Banana Muffins

Irish Oatmeal

How to cook Irish Oats the night before:

1 cup Irish Oats
4 cups water

Before bed bring to a boil for 5 minutes. Turn off stove and let sit overnight. In the morning you will have 4 servings of perfectly cooked oatmeal.

Oatmeal with Warm Banana

1 cup cooked Irish oats
2 egg whites
½ sliced Banana
Splash of skim milk

Combine all ingredients well and warm in the microwave for 2 to 3 minutes.

1 serving

Calories	Carbohydrates	Fat	Protein	Fiber
246	42	2.9	13.9	5.5

Strawberry Banana Breakfast Bonanza

¾ cup plain 0% plain Greek yogurt
½ cup Kashi Go Lean Crunch
2 ounces chopped banana
2 ounces sliced strawberry

Serve and Enjoy!

* It's like dessert for breakfast but healthy and full of calcium and protein! It's got everything you need to start your day off right.

Calories	Carbohydrates	Fat	Protein	Fiber
294	43.7	1.9	26.2	7.1

No Toast French Toast

Serves 1

Well, it doesn't look like French toast, but it sure tastes like it.

3 egg whites
A dash of cinnamon (to your taste)
A splash of vanilla (to your taste)

1) Whip your egg whites as if you were making meringue. But don't make meringue. Whip them until they are triple in size. They should definitely be fluffy, but not hard.
2) Fold in your cinnamon and vanilla.
3) Spray a pan with olive oil and heat on medium. Slowly pour your fluffy whites on the pan. (They should be about an inch high, not flat and runny.) Let them cook on medium/low for at least five minutes. When you're confident the bottom is cooked and ready to flip, flip and cook the other side.

You can eat this as is. You can add fresh berries. You can even add a touch of pure maple syrup.

As is-

Calories	Carbohydrates	Protein	Fat	Fiber
58	1.8	10.8	.2	.6

Cinnamon French Toast

2 slices of Ezekiel Cinnamon Bread, defrosted
3 egg whites
Dash of cinnamon
Dash of vanilla
½ banana
Canola oil spray

1) Heat both pans on medium.
2) Whisk egg whites, cinnamon and vanilla in a bowl.
3) Drench your Ezekiel bread in your egg mixture.
4) Spray both your pans with a touch of oil.
5) In one pan: place your toast and top it off with any remaining egg. Then brown both sides!
6) In the other pan – sauté your sliced banana
7) Place your banana on-top of your French toast and voila!

Calories	Carbohydrates	Protein	Fat	Fiber
275	50.1	17.4	1.7	5.5

Popeye Pancakes

Makes 8-10.

3 egg whites—whip until they *almost* start to form peeks

In a bowl combine:
½ cup oat bran
½ cup whole wheat flour
1 tsp baking powder
½ tsp cinnamon

Add to your bowl:
1 ½ cups low-fat cottage cheese
1 Tbsp maple syrup
¼ cup Greek yogurt

Slowly fold in whipped egg whites

1) Spray a pan with olive oil and set it to medium.
2) Drop 2 Tbsp of batter on greased pan to form a pancake.
3) Cook on both sides and serve!

- Note: Once your spatula gets batter on it, the pancakes get harder and harder to flip. Keep a napkin handy to frequently clean off your spatula.

A Great Topping:

1) Slice a very ripe banana into thin pieces.
2) Heat a pan on medium and spray with olive oil.
3) Sauté banana until it is lightly brown.
4) Serve over pancakes!

1 Pancake

Calories	Carbohydrates	Protein	Fat	Fiber
78	10.7	7.7	.9	1.7

Salsa Omelet

4 egg whites
A touch of skim milk
Diced onion
Red peppers
Salsa
Sliced avocado (approximately 1 ounce)
A sprinkle of low-fat shredded cheddar cheese (½ ounce)
Salt and pepper to taste

1) Whisk together your eggs, salt, pepper and a touch of milk. Set aside.
2) Spray a pan with olive oil. Sauté your onions and peppers on medium.
3) Remove the veggies from your pan and re-spray.
4) Add your egg mixture to the pan and allow it to cook until the sides begin to lift.
5) Once the bottom is cooked, flip.
6) Place already cooked veggies in the middle of your eggs along with a tablespoon of your favorite salsa, avocado and a sprinkle of cheese.
7) Close it up. Give the cheese a minute to melt and serve.

1 omelet

Calories	Carbohydrates	Protein	Fat	Fiber
178	7.5	22.4	6.4	2.7

Goat Cheese Omelet

4 egg whites
A touch of skim milk
Diced onion
Garlic, mashed
Baby spinach (½ cup)
Fresh diced tomatoes
Salt and Pepper to taste
Goat cheese. (½ ounce)

1) Whisk your eggs, salt, pepper and a touch of milk together in a bowl.
2) Spray a pan with olive oil and cook your onions, garlic, spinach and fresh tomatoes on medium.
3) Remove the veggies from your pan and re-spray.
4) Add your egg mixture to the pan and allow it to cook on medium until the sides begin to lift. Once the bottom is cooked, flip.
5) Place your already cooked veggies in middle of your eggs. Close it up.
6) Spread your goat cheese on top and serve.

*A little goes a long way when you can see the cheese. Who knows why, but I think I taste it more when I see it.

1 omelet

Calories	Carbohydrates	Protein	Fat	Fiber
143	6	18.9	4.7	1.4

Egg White and Feta Quesadilla

1 small whole grain tortilla
3 egg whites
6 cheery tomatoes, diced
1 ounce crumbled feta cheese

1) On medium, spray pan with olive oil and sauté tomatoes until they are soft and cooked.
2) Remove tomatoes from pan. In the same pan, scramble egg whites.
3) Remove whites. Place quesadilla in already warm pan.
4) Top one half with eggs, tomatoes and feta.
5) Fold and brown on both sides.

1 Quesadilla

Calories	Carbohydrates	Protein	Fat	Fiber
245	17.6	19	10.2	3.4

Bacon, Swiss and Asparagus Frittata

Oven at 350. Serves 4

I like to make this frittata and have it for lunch. Great for leftovers! It will keep in your fridge for several days, but it does not freeze well.

In a pan;
1 Tbsp margarine
1 leek, diced
1 cup fat-free milk
2 garlic cloves, mashed
1 tsp nutmeg

In a bowl:
6 egg whites
3 eggs
1 cup asparagus spears, steamed and chopped
3 pieces cooked Canadian bacon, chopped
2 ounces light Swiss, grated
1 Tbsp Dijon mustard
3-4 chives, chopped
Salt and pepper to taste

1) On medium heat, melt margarine; sauté leeks and garlic.
2) Add milk and nutmeg to the pan. Bring to a boil, and then simmer on low 7-10 minutes.
3) Allow the mixture to cool.

In a bowl:

1) Whisk egg whites and eggs together.
2) Stir in asparagus, turkey bacon, Swiss cheese, mustard, chives, salt and pepper. Combine well.
3) Pour in cooled milk mixture.
4) Spray a pie plate with olive oil and pour your egg mixture in.

Bake at 350 for 45 minutes.

2 slices

Calories	Carbohydrates	Protein	Fat	Fiber
184	8	18.5	7.7	1.1

Vegetable and Cheese Crust-less Quiche

Oven at 350. Serves 4

In a pan:
1 Tbsp margarine
1 small onion, diced
1 cup sliced mushrooms
1 ½ cups broccoli florets, chopped
1 zucchini, grated
2 garlic cloves, mashed
1 cup nonfat milk
½ tsp nutmeg

1) Melt margarine in a pan and sauté diced onions, mushrooms and garlic.
2) Once the onions become soft and clear add broccoli and zucchini.
3) Add milk.
4) Bring to a boil and then simmer on low for 7-10 minutes.
5) Sprinkle nutmeg and let cool.

In a bowl:
6 egg whites
3 eggs
1 ounce Parmesan & 1 ounce sharp cheddar cheese, grated
Salt and pepper to taste (the cheese is already salty so you don't need much)

1) Whisk your egg whites and eggs together in a bowl.
2) Stir in your cheese and milk mixture.
3) Spray a pie plate with olive oil spray and pour in your eggs.

Bake at 350 for 45 minutes.

2 slices

Calories	Carbohydrates	Protein	Fat	Fiber
192	10.5	16.9	9.4	2.4

Eggs Jenny

This one is so easy and so delicious!

3 egg whites
1 slice Canadian Bacon (1 ounce)
1 slice sprouted grain bread (or whatever you choose. You can even make this a wrap)
1 slice low-fat cheddar cheese (1 ounce)

1) Cook bacon in a pan on medium. Remove.
2) Without cleaning your pan, cook your egg whites.
3) Place your cheese on your bread and toast it to melt the cheese.
4) On top of your cheese toast, layer your bacon and eggs.

* Feel free to close this sandwich with a second piece of bread!

Calories	Carbohydrates	Protein	Fat	Fiber
233	16.6	28.6	5	3

Peanut Butter Banana Chocolate Breakfast Cookies

Oven at 350. Makes 18.

I have friends offering to pay me money to make these bad boys for them. I love to make a big batch and freeze them. They last forever (if you don't give in to the temptation to eat three in a row). For a "cookie," these are high in protein and fiber. Great for breakfast on the go with a piece of fruit. Or try them as a snack in the middle of the day.

In a bowl, combine:
2 cups Old Fashioned rolled oats
½ cup & 2 Tbsp whole wheat flour
2 Tbsp ground flax
1 tsp of baking powder
2 tsp cinnamon
Salt to taste

In another bowl, blend together:
3 egg whites
1/3 cup brown sugar
2 very ripe bananas, mashed
¼ cup natural peanut butter
4 Mission figs, mashed to a pulp
2 tsp vanilla
* I use a hand mixer to make sure I really break up and mash the figs.

Combine dry and wet bowls together.

ADD:

   1) Ghirardelli 60% dark chocolate chips (4 servings; about 64 chips)
   2) 1/3 cup chopped walnut pieces
      1. Drop cookies onto a greased sheet.
      2. Bake at 350 for 25 minutes.

1 cookie

Calories	Carbohydrates	Protein	Fat	Fiber
134	18.1	4.2	5.5	3

Cinnamon Apple bombs!

Makes 16. Oven at 350.

<u>In a bowl, combine:</u>
1 cup of bran buds cereal
1 cup of skim milk
* Let the mixture sit until it forms a nice mush.
   If you're impatient, blend it with a hand blender

<u>In another bowl, combine:</u>
2/3 cup whole wheat flour
1 ½ cups oat bran
1 ½ tsp baking powder
½ tsp baking soda
1 tsp all spice
1 tsp salt
1 heaping tsp cinnamon

<u>In another bowl, puree with a blender:</u>
1/3 cup brown sugar
1 egg white
1 large apple, peeled & chopped
Pitted prunes (4), mashed to a pulp (or 1 container of prune baby food)
2 Tbsp Greek style 0% yogurt

Once your bran mixture is soaked, mix all three bowls together. Combine well.

Add:
1 cup raisins
1 large apple (peeled and cut into small cubes)

Pour batter into small muffin tins.
* Do not use paper tins as there is not enough oil in these muffins and they will stick to the paper.
   Either spray your tins with olive oil or use silicon muffin cups.

Bake at 350 for 28 minutes

1 muffin

Calories	Carbohydrates	Protein	Fat	Fiber
90	21	2.7	.7	4.2

5 Banana Banana Muffins

Oven at 350. Makes 24

In a Bowl- Combine:
1 cup whole wheat flour
1 cup oat flour
½ cup oat bran
1 ½ tsp baking powder
1 tsp baking soda

In another bowl, puree with a blender (I use a handheld):
16 Mission figs, diced
2 egg whites
1 ½ tsp vanilla
1 cup unsweetened applesauce
5 very ripe bananas

Combine both bowls together and mix well.

Add:
- 4 servings Ghirardelli 60% Dark Chocolate chips (62 chips)
- ½ cup chopped walnuts

Pour batter into small muffin tins.
*Do not use paper tins as there is not enough oil in these muffins and they will stick to the paper. Either spray your tins with olive oil or use silicon muffin cups.

Bake at 350 for 35 minutes.

1 muffin

Calories	Carbohydrates	Protein	Fat	Fiber
114	10.2	2.7	3.6	3.1

Snack Ideas

I post a list of snacks I have in my house on the fridge door. I never open the fridge door without knowing what I'm going in there for.

* Fresh cut-up veggies
Any veggies you have in the house.
When I get home from the grocery store the first thing I do is cut up the veggies that I have bought into munch-able strips. I put them in a container full of water so that they keep longer and they are there ready for me to grab when I need them.

* Celery and peanut butter or whole grain crackers (like Wasa) and peanut butter.
  1 Tbsp of P.B and some fresh cut celery.

* 0% Greek yogurt and fresh or frozen berries.

* A serving of low fat cheese.

* Toasted raw nuts (1 ounce)
WARNING: Nuts are a great snack. If you're like me, you can eat them like candy! Make sure you measure out your one-ounce serving and put the rest away. I split up my nuts into mini sandwich bags when I get home from the market.

* The Laughing Cow light cheese
Sometimes I spread this on a piece of sprouted grain bread with a slice of tomato and fresh basil.

* ½ cup boiled edamame
Sometimes I sprinkle popcorn seasoning on these. It tastes like I'm eating flavored chips!

* ½ cup low-fat cottage cheese with cinnamon
Or with fresh berries

* A glass of fat-free milk

* A ½ glass of fat-free milk with ½ cup of low-fat chocolate milk

* 2 cups fresh popped popcorn

* Fruit smoothie
½ cup yogurt, ¼ cup milk, frozen berries and blend!

* Any piece of fresh fruit

* A green apple with an ounce of sliced fresh Parmesan

* Wasa crackers with light Swiss cheese

* 1 slice of whole grain toast with 1 Tbsp Almond Butter or Cashew Butter

* Banana slices with 1 Tbsp peanut butter

* Boiled egg whites with hummus
At the beginning of the week I will boil four to six eggs. I keep them in the fridge. When it's snack time, I simply remove the yolk and replace it with hummus!

* Gnu Bar * Lara Bar * A Simply Bar

The reason I love these bars so much is that they are preservative-free. Made with whole foods, there is nothing on the label I cannot understand.

My favorite meal—pizza!

I am so excited to share. This recipe was passed down to me from a good friend.

3 egg whites
1 serving turkey pepperoni
2 Tbsp marinara sauce
4 button mushrooms, sliced
Dash of oregano
Sprinkle of low-fat Mozzarella (1/2 ounce)

1) Place turkey pepperoni in an unsprayed frying pan on high. Sauté.
2) Stir in your diced mushrooms and a dash of oregano.
3) Once turkey is cooked to your liking (I like mine crispy) remove from pan.
4) Spray your pan (no need to clean it) with olive oil.
5) Re-add the turkey and mushroom mixture. Pour your egg whites on top.
6) Once the sides of your eggs begin to lift, flip. Try hard to keep a round shape. If it looks like a pizza, it's bound to taste like a pizza!
7) Spread your marinara sauce on top and sprinkle with cheese.
8) Lower your heat and allow your cheese to melt. Serve.

You can add anything to this pizza. My husband likes to add pineapple chunks.

1 Pizza

Calories	Carbohydrates	Protein	Fat	Fiber
198	7.1	25.8	6.8	1.7

Ideas for packing a Lunch

* Make a sandwich! Bring an apple, and a cheese string.
* Throw leftovers from dinner in a container.
* Bring a container of home made soup, heat it in the microwave along with a sandwich.
* Bring a cold cooked chicken breast and a bag of lettuce. Toss at work!
* Bring a container of homemade chili.
* Make a pizza with a whole grain pita! Wrap it in tinfoil.
* Make a wrap and bring it along with a piece of fruit.
* Make a batch of couscous or quinoa. Both are delicious at room temperature.
* Always remember to pack one or two healthy snacks with your lunch.

Sandwiches

I don't know why everyone forgot how good sandwiches really are. There is nothing wrong with a healthy sandwich on whole grain bread.

Peanut Butter and Banana

Bacon, Cheddar and Tomato

My Fav'wich

My Hubby's Fav'wich

Tuna Salad

Tuna Melt

Chicken Curry with Fruit Chutney

Peanut Butter and Banana

This is one I crave! A peanut butter sandwich and a glass of cold milk!
I make mine with:

2 slices sprouted grain bread, toasted
1 Tbsp natural peanut butter
1 ½ ounces sliced banana

1 Sandwich

Calories	Carbohydrates	Protein	Fat	Fiber
283	42.7	10	9.6	6.6

Bacon, Cheddar and Tomato

2 slices sprouted grain, toasted
1 slice Canadian Back Bacon (1 ounce)
1 slice low-fat Cheddar cheese (1 ounce)
Tomato slices

1 Sandwich

Calories	Carbohydrates	Protein	Fat	Fiber
267	32.1	22	5.4	6.4

My Fav'wich

Serves 2

1 whole grain baguette (4 ounces) cut in half, keeping one side of bread attached.
* Baguettes tend to be big, so make sure to look at how many servings are in the loaf.

Remove most of the insides of the bread. (You want to taste the sandwich not the bread.) Sorry, getting excited just writing this one down!

Then I spread:
2 wedges of The Laughing Cow Light Swiss cheese
1 Tbsp low-sugar apricot preserves on top of the cheese
½ green apple, thinly sliced
4 ounces sliced nitrate free turkey meat
Close, cut and serve!

1 Sandwich

Calories	Carbohydrates	Protein	Fat	Fiber
312	51.7	18.3	4	4.6

My Hubby's Fav'wich

2 slices sprouted grain, toasted
2 ounces sliced nitrate free turkey meat
1 ounce avocado, sliced
Honey mustard
1 large dill pickle, sliced. (Yes, put the pickle in the sandwich!)

1 Sandwich

Calories	Carbohydrates	Protein	Fat	Fiber
266	38.5	16.6	6.2	7

Tuna Salad

Serves 2

1 can Albacore tuna in water
2 large Tbsp 0% Greek style yogurt
1 tsp honey Dijon mustard
Salt and pepper to taste

Mix!

To this mixture add:

Option A) Chopped pickles, splash of Apple Cider vinegar.

Option B) Chopped green olives, splash of Apple Cider vinegar.

Option C) Chopped green or red apple, splash of Balsamic vinegar.

Option D) Chopped celery and almonds, splash of Balsamic vinegar.

Per Serving (with pickles)

Calories	Carbohydrates	Protein	Fat	Fiber
98	2.9	17.5	1.1	.6

Open Faced Tuna Melt

Make an open faced tuna melt with one of the above options:

1) Toast two pieces of whole grain or sprouted grain bread.
2) Add the tuna mixture on top and lightly sprinkle with low-fat cheddar cheese (¼ of a cup, divided).

Place back in toaster oven to melt to cheese.

1 melt. (2 slices)

Calories	Carbohydrates	Protein	Fat	Fiber
293	34.9	30.5	4.1	4.8

Curry Chicken Salad with Fruit Chutney

Serves 4

2 Tbsp of any kind of low-sugar fruit chutney or jam preserves
Wasa crackers (or whole grain toast)

10 ounces chopped white meat chicken
2 very heaping Tbsp 0% Greek yogurt (to whatever creaminess you desire)
1 ½ tsp lemon juice
1 ½ tsp curry powder
Dash of ground ginger
Dash of cinnamon
2 ounces of Craisins
Sprinkle of fresh green onions
Salt and pepper to taste

1) Chop chicken and add to it: yogurt, lemon juice and spices.
2) Combine well.
3) Season with salt and pepper.
4) Spread jam on a Wasa or toast.
   • Strawberry or Cranberry are both really good.
5) Lightly top with curry chicken and a sprinkle of green onions.

1 serving on 2 Wasa crackers

Calories	Carbohydrates	Protein	Fat	Fiber
266	36.4	28.3	2.2	5.2

A note about chicken

Having cooked chicken in the house is a great way to make meal times really simple. You can use it in salads, wraps, sandwiches, stir fries or on its own.

Here are a couple of ways I keep cooked chicken in my fridge.

1) Buy a pre-cooked rotisserie chicken.
2) Marinate and grill a bunch of chicken breasts for the week.
3) Boil chicken breasts in low-sodium chicken broth and keep them in the fridge.

Chicken Wrap

Mexican Chicken Wrap

Caesar Wrap

Buffalo Wing Wrap

Asian Wrap

Easy Chicken Salad

Chopped Chicken Salad

Chicken Parmesan

Corn Flake Chicken

Turkey Schnitzel

Greek Chicken Skewers

Roast Turkey Breast

Turkey Schnitzel

Chicken Wraps

Wraps can be whatever you want them to be. They are easy, delicious and healthy!

For a supper healthy option, you can use lettuce as your wrap. Butter lettuce works great. You can also use a whole grain wrap or pita.
Here is the 'wrap' breakdown:

Type	Calories	Carbohydrates	Protein	Fat	Fiber
Generic Whole Wheat Wrap	120	16	2	5	2
Generic Whole Wheat Pita	140	27	6	1.5	4
Butter Lettuce Leaf	2	0.3	0.2	0	0.2

Chicken Wrap:

Use 3 to 4 ounces of white meat rotisserie chicken
Diced tomatoes
Avocado
Lettuce (if it's not already being used as a wrap)
1 Tbsp fat-free Italian dressing or ½ Tbsp BBQ sauce

Without an actual wrap

Calories	Carbohydrates	Protein	Fat	Fiber
205	12.8	25.9	9.6	5.5

Mexican Chicken Wrap:

Use 3 to 4 ounces white meat chicken
¼ cup black beans
1 Tbsp 0% Greek yogurt or low-fat sour cream
Salsa
Avocado
Lettuce (if it's not already being used as a wrap)

Without an actual wrap

Calories	Carbohydrates	Protein	Fat	Fiber
260	21.4	31.8	8.8	8.1

Caesar Wrap:

Dust your chicken in this:
Cajun spice mix (Emerald's Essence is great!)

Or marinate your chicken in Frank's Hot Wing Sauce.
Or use rotisserie.

Use 3-4 ounces white meat chicken
1 slice cooked turkey bacon
1 Tbsp grated Parmesan cheese
1 Tbsp light Caesar dressing
Diced tomatoes
Chopped romaine lettuce

Without an actual wrap

Calories	Carbohydrates	Protein	Fat	Fiber
212	3.1	27.8	9.8	0

Buffalo Wing Wrap:

3-4 ounces white meat chicken marinated in Frank's Hot Wing Sauce
Diced tomatoes
Diced lettuce
1 Tbsp light blue cheese dressing
Avocado
Shredded carrots
Celery pieces

Without an actual wrap

Calories	Carbohydrates	Protein	Fat	Fiber
202	7.2	24.2	8	2.6

Asian Style Wrap:

3-4 ounces white meat chicken
Handful of shredded carrots
Handful of shredded cabbage
1 Tbsp light sesame ginger salad dressing
Tangerine slices
Sprinkle of toasted almonds, sliced (1 tbsp)

Without an actual wrap

Calories	Carbohydrates	Protein	Fat	Fiber
231	14	25.8	7.9	2.7

Easy Chicken Salad

Buy a pre-cooked rotisserie chicken from the store.

1) Buy a bag of lettuce from the store.
2) Use your favorite low-fat dressing (or make your own).
3) Toss and serve.

Sprinkle on some nuts and add a little dried fruit if you've got it! Be inventive, it's the easiest meal around.

3-ounce chicken breast, low-fat dressing and lettuce

Calories	Carbohydrates	Protein	Fat	Fiber
163	9.2	21.4	5.4	2.7

Chopped Chicken Salad

Makes 4 servings.

I normally use the chicken meat I have left over from making a pot of chicken soup for my chopped chicken salad. (I must confess, I combine dark and white meat)

If you haven't just made a fresh pot, you can always go straight to my good old favorite, rotisserie chicken.

Chopped chicken, 11 ounces (give or take)
2 very heaping Tbsp of 0% Greek style yogurt (add more if you like it creamier)
1 flat Tbsp of honey Dijon mustard
1 ounce toasted almonds, diced and chopped
1 ½ tsp lime juice
3-4 pickles, diced

1) On large cutting board: Dice chicken. Squirt with lemon juice and add to it yogurt and mustard.
2) Blend and dice well.
3) Add chopped almonds and diced pickles. Blend and chop.
* You can add whatever you like to this instead of the pickles and almonds.

Per Serving

Calories	Carbohydrates	Protein	Fat	Fiber
234	8.1	21.7	12.8	2.1

Baked Chicken Parmesan

Serves 4. Oven at 350.

3 Tbsp almond meal (heaping)
3 Tbsp whole wheat flour (heaping)
3 Tbsp Panko Crumbs (heaping)
1 Tbsp paprika
1 tsp mustard powder
1 tsp garlic salt
2 tsp onion powder
1 egg
8 Tbsp marinara sauce
4 Tbsp grated Parmesan cheese
4 chicken breasts

1) On a large plate, combine almond meal, whole wheat flour and spices.
2) Whisk egg in a bowl and dunk your chicken breasts in.
3) Coat chicken with the almond meal mixture.
4) Place on sprayed cookie sheet and bake for 20-25 minutes.
5) Remove chicken from oven. Cover each piece with 2 Tbsp marinara and 1 Tbsp Parmesan cheese.
6) Broil on high for 5 minutes, or until cheese bubbles.

3.5-ounce chicken breast

Calories	Carbohydrates	Protein	Fat	Fiber
281	12.6	36.7	8.7	2.1

Greek Chicken Skewers with Tzatziki

Serves 4

4 chicken breasts cut into cubes

Marinate chicken cubes overnight in:
6 Tbsp lemon juice
2 Tbsp red wine vinegar
½ cup fat-free Italian salad dressing
5 garlic cloves, mashed
1 Tbsp dried oregano
1 Tbsp dried rosemary
1 Tbsp dried thyme
Salt and pepper to taste

Marinate vegetables for at least 1 hour in fat-free Italian dressing:
Green pepper, cut into 1-inch pieces
Red pepper, cut into 1-inch pieces
Red onion, cut into 1-inch pieces
Zucchini, cut into 1-inch pieces

1) Soak wood skewers for 20 minutes in a water bath.
2) Place well-marinated chicken on skewers interlaced with vegetables.
3) BBQ on medium until chicken is cooked through.
4) Serve with Tzatziki.

You can also serve with my Greek Salad! The marinade and dressing are very similar so it's easy to make them together.

3.5-ounce chicken breast with grilled veggies

Calories	Carbohydrates	Protein	Fat	Fiber
184	4.5	31.6	3.7	1.1

Cornflake Chicken

So easy. So delicious. Oven at 350.

Chicken breasts
Fat-free Italian salad dressing (enough to marinate chicken in)
Cornflake crumbs

1) Poke chicken breasts with a fork to make several holes.
2) Marinate your chicken breast in fat-free Italian salad dressing at least 1 hour; overnight is best.
3) Coat breasts in corn flake crumbs and place bake for 20-25 minutes.

3.5-ounce chicken breast

Calories	Carbohydrates	Protein	Fat	Fiber
211	10.8	31.8	3.5	.1

Turkey Schnitzel

Serves 4

16 ounces Turkey Scalopini (Thinly sliced raw boneless skinless turkey breasts)
1 large lemon
1 Tbsp. olive oil
1 egg
3 Tbsp (heaping) almond meal
3 Tbsp (heaping) whole-wheat flour
1 tsp garlic powder
1tsp mustard powder
2 Tbsp fresh parsley
Salt and pepper to taste

1) Spray a frying pan with olive oil spray and set to medium on your stovetop.
2) In a bowl combine almond meal, spices, whole-wheat flour and parsley.
3) In another bowl beat egg.
4) Dip your turkey in the egg and coat in the almond meal mixture.
5) Cook on stove stop; 3- 4 minutes a side.
6) Serve with a slice of lemon.

Calories	Carbohydrates	Protein	Fat	Fiber
185	6.9	30.6	5.6	3.3

Roast Turkey Breast with Vegetables

Serves 4. Oven at 325.

2 ½ -3 lb turkey breast

1) Place turkey breast in roasting pan lined with foil.
2) Spread a variety of vegetables around your turkey. I use:
   2 baby red potatoes, halved
   1 large sweet potato, peeled and cut into cubes
   8 small Brussels sprouts
   1 large carrot, cut into pieces
   1 parsnip, cut into pieces
   1 onion, quartered and peeled.
3) Fold foil up to cup vegetables and keep juices in.
4) Season breast with:
   Salt and pepper to taste
   1 Tbsp paprika
   2 Tbsp olive oil
   2 Tbsp maple syrup
   2 tsp garlic powder
   ½ cup chicken broth
5) Bake for 1 hour, basting at the 30-minute mark.
6) Remove from oven: pour in additional 1 cup chicken broth.
7) Bake for approximately another 45 minutes (baste halfway).
8) Thermometer should read 160 when turkey is done.

3.5-ounces turkey, potatoes and vegetables

Calories	Carbohydrates	Protein	Fat	Fiber
366	36.2	32.4	10.1	5

You can also find "ready to cook from frozen" turkey breast in your grocers freezer. Just follow the directions and serve!

Stir Fry Recipes

Whip up an easy stir-fry. Choose a protein, open a bag of frozen veggies, stir, sauce, and serve with ½ cup of brown rice! Want to know how I like to season mine?

2 Tbsp natural peanut butter
2 Tbsp low-sodium soy sauce

Or

½ cup low-sodium chicken broth
1 minced garlic clove
Dash of fresh ginger (or ½ tsp powder)
1 tsp low sodium soy
2 tsp rice vinegar
¼ tsp sesame oil

Ground Turkey

Oh, what I can do with a package of lean ground turkey. I buy four at a time and freeze them. They come in so handy. Here are my staples.

Turkey Burgers

Greek Turkey Burgers

Meatloaf by Mistake

Spaghetti Squash with Turkey Bolognaise

No Noodle Lasagna

My Baby's Chili

Thai Lettuce Wraps

Turkey Burgers

Makes 8 Burgers

These are great for the BBQ. But if it's not BBQ season, they can easily be made on the stovetop. Either way they are delicious.

I like to dress these burgers with sliced dill pickles and tomatoes.

1 package lean ground turkey (20 ounces)
1/3 cup old fashioned oatmeal flakes
1 small onion, diced
1 egg
1½ Tbsp of honey Dijon mustard
2 ½ Tbsp Worchester sauce
2 Tbsp Barbeque Sauce

1) Blend all ingredients well.
2) Form 3-4 oz burgers (8 burgers).
3) BBQ on medium. OR cook on medium on your stovetop.
4) In both cases, spray with olive oil.

One Burger. (Recipe makes 8)

Calories	Carbohydrates	Protein	Fat	Fiber
166	7.9	19.4	6.5	.6

Try these on an Ezekiel sprouted grain or whole wheat bun!

Greek Style Turkey Burgers

Makes 8 Burgers.

1 package lean ground turkey meat
½ medium onion, diced
2 garlic cloves, mashed
1 Tbsp Dijon mustard
½ cup oat bran
¼ cup black olives, diced
¼ cup sun dried tomatoes, diced
2 oz crumbled light feta cheese
2 Tbsp Italian salad dressing
1 egg, whisked

1) Combine all ingredients and divide into 4 oz burgers patties.
2) BBQ and enjoy! Great with a side of Tzatziki.

4 ounce Burger

Calories	Carbohydrates	Protein	Fat	Fiber
183	7.1	18.1	8.4	1.3

Meatloaf by Mistake

Makes 6 servings. Oven to 350.

TOPPING
1 Tbsp olive oil
1 small onion, diced
1 cup mushrooms, sliced
½ red pepper, diced
½ green pepper, diced
2 garlic cloves, mashed

1) Heat oil on medium.
2) Sauté onions, mushrooms and garlic for 5 minutes.
3) Add peppers. Vegetables should be soft, not brown. Set aside.

LOAF
1 package lean ground turkey meat
1 egg, beaten
1 small onion, diced
1 ½ cup marinara sauce (store-bought or homemade)
2 Tbsp honey Dijon mustard
Salt and pepper to taste
½ cup of Steel Cut Irish oats, uncooked

1) In a mixing bowl, beat egg.
2) Add marinara, mustard and onions. Blend.
3) Mix in turkey and oats.
4) Salt and pepper to taste.
5) Spray a loaf pan with olive oil and place meat mixture in your pan.
6) Cover the top of your meat mixture with the cooked vegetable mixture.
7) Bake at 350 for 90 minutes.

* *Let sit for 1 hour before serving.*

1 of 6

Calories	Carbohydrates	Protein	Fat	Fiber
269	17.5	23.3	10.6	2.9

Spaghetti Squash with Turkey Bolognaise

There are many things you can do with spaghetti squash. In my house, we use it to replace pasta a lot.

The Spaghetti

1) Cut your spaghetti squash in half and remove the seeds.
2) Place one half in a microwavable dish (covered, flat side up.) with a ½ inch of water for 12-15 minutes.
3) Repeat with other half.
4) Once the squash has cooled, pull at it with a fork and it will come apart like spaghetti.
5) Place the spaghetti in a colander and let sit for five minutes. (This will drain any excess water.)

1 cup

Calories	Carbohydrates	Protein	Fat	Fiber
39	9.3	1	.4	2

The Meat for the Sauce
1 package lean ground turkey (20 ounces)
Season with:
½ Tbsp of mustard
2 Tbsp Worcestershire sauce
1 small onion, diced.
1 cup Marinara sauce
Montreal Steak Spice to taste

1) Blend well.
2) Cook in a pan on medium/high heat, making sure the meat crumbles.

1 of 6 servings

Calories	Carbohydrates	Protein	Fat	Fiber
169	4.9	19.9	7	.7

No Noodle Lasagna

Serves 8. Oven at 325.

1 package spicy or sweet lean turkey sausages.
1 cup tomato pasta sauce
2 Tbsp tomato paste
1 Tbsp of olive oil
½ small onion, diced
½ red pepper, diced
½ cup mushrooms, diced
2 garlic cloves, mashed
1 Tbsp basil
1 Tbsp oregano

8 ounces light Ricotta cheese
3 egg whites beaten
Salt and pepper to taste
Fresh parsley

¼ cup Parmesan cheese, grated
½ cup 2% shredded Mozzarella cheese

2 medium zucchinis cut thinly lengthwise (they will be your noodles!)
½ bag baby spinach (steamed)

1) Heat a pan with olive oil. Sauté onions, spices and zucchini strips until onions soften and zucchini strips are seared. Remove zucchini strips and set aside.
2) Remove sausage meat from casings and cook together with onions and spices. Brown and crumble.
3) Add peppers and mushrooms.
4) Pour in tomato sauce and tomato paste.

1) Beat egg whites and Ricotta together in a bowl.
2) Add chopped fresh parsley, salt and pepper.

1) Spray a casserole dish with olive oil.
2) Spread ½ of the meat mixture on the bottom of the dish.
3) Top with thinly sliced zucchini to cover meat.
4) Top zucchini with ½ ricotta mixture.
5) Top ricotta mixture with ½ steamed spinach.
6) Top spinach with ½ mozzarella.
7) Repeat.
8) After the last layer of mozzarella, finish off with Parmesan cheese.

Bake at 325 for 45 minutes or until cheese is bubbly and golden.
Broil for 5 minutes.
Let sit for 45 minutes-1 hour before you serve.

1 slice of 8

Calories	Carbohydrates	Protein	Fat	Fiber
215	7.2	19.8	12.7	1.5

My Baby's Chili

Makes 7 servings.

1 small onion diced
2 garlic cloves mashed
1 Tbsp olive oil
1 package lean ground turkey meat
1 can diced tomatoes (14.5 ounces)
1 Tbsp tomato paste
1 tsp vanilla extract
1 Tbsp brown sugar
1 Tbsp Worcestershire sauce
1 small can kidney beans
2 small sweet potatoes, peeled and cubed
1 ½ Tbsp chili powder
Salt and pepper to taste
Low-fat shredded Cheddar cheese

1) In a large saucepan, heat olive oil. Soften onions and garlic.
2) Add turkey and season with salt and pepper.
3) As turkey begins to brown add chili powder.
4) Pour in tomatoes, tomato paste, vanilla, brown sugar and Worcestershire.
5) Add sweet potatoes and beans. Mix Well.
6) Let simmer on low for 1 hour or until potatoes are cooked through.

Sprinkle each serving with 1 Tbsp low-fat shredded cheddar cheese.

1 serving

Calories	Carbohydrates	Protein	Fat	Fiber
231	19.8	19.7	8.1	4.4

Thai Lettuce Wraps with Ground Turkey

Makes 4-5 servings.

1 package lean ground turkey
2 Tbsp Hoisin sauce
3 Tbsp Thai Sweet Chili sauce
1 cup water chestnuts, sliced
1 Tbsp olive oil
Salt and pepper to taste

Butter Lettuce Heads

1) Heat olive oil in a pan on medium/high heat.
2) Add ground turkey and season with salt and pepper, making sure turkey crumbles as it cooks.
3) Add Hoisin and Chili sauce. Simmer until your meat is cooked.
4) Toss in water chestnuts.

Make a wrap! Spoon your turkey meat into a leaf of butter lettuce! Top with:

Shredded carrots
Tangerine slices
Bean sprouts
Toasted Almonds
Angel hair noodles

3.5 ounces Turkey Meat

Calories	Carbohydrates	Protein	Fat	Fiber
157.5	7.7	15	6.8	.6

Pasta and Noodles

Now, I know people who "diet" think pasta is off limits. It's not. You just have to have it in moderation.

Most noodles have a serving size of ¾ of a cup or 2 oz.

Measure out one serving in the bowl you are actually going to eat it in to help you familiarize yourself with a serving. Adding lots veggies and protein is the key to healthy, delicious and filling pasta.

Shirataki noodles

Fusilli Pesto Pasta

Veggie Pasta with Tomato Sauce

Peanut Butter Goodness

Shirataki KD style

Shirataki noodles.

You will find these in the tofu section at your local grocery store. Don't let these guys scare you. They are a great low-fat, low-calorie option.

They come in a sealed package floating in water. When you're ready to use them, cut the package open and place noodles in a strainer. Rinse well with water and pat dry with a paper towel. Use them as you would use already cooked noodles. You can find them in a variety of styles: Fettuccini, Angel Hair and Spaghetti.

They have a similar texture to an egg noodle, or a noodle you would find in chicken soup. They are softer then pasta. But they are delicious and worth a try, I promise. There are quick and easy recipes on the back of the package.

- *2 oz of Whole Grain Pasta runs you at least 200 calories, 42 carbohydrates and 2 grams of fiber.*

Tofu Shirataki Noodles – per serving 2 oz serving

Calories	Carbohydrates	Protein	Fat	Fiber
20	3	1	.5	2

Fusilli Pesto Pasta

Serves 4

8 oz whole grain pasta.
** *You can also make this dish with* <u>*Shirataki noodles*</u>—*it will cut calories and carbohydrates dramatically!*
1 ounce toasted pine nuts, divided into 4 servings
¼ cup pesto
2 garlic cloves, mashed
1 cup asparagus, trimmed and diced
1 medium zucchini, sliced
½ cup cherry tomatoes, cut in half
8 oz chicken breast, cooked and chopped
Salt and pepper to taste
4 Tbsp grated Parmesan cheese, separated into 4 servings

1) Boil noodles as directed. (I like them al dante). Drain and set aside.
2) Spray a large pan with olive oil. Add garlic, zucchini, and asparagus.
3) Once veggies have softened, add cooked chicken and tomatoes. Season with salt and pepper to taste.
4) Pour in pesto and toss to coat.
5) Toss in cooked noodles and pine nuts. Stir, serve and top with cheese.

One serving

Calories	Carbohydrates	Protein	Fat	Fiber
442	48.6	31	14.8	6.9

Veggie Pasta with Tomato Sauce

Serves 4

8 oz whole grain penne
2 cups marinara sauce. *Approximately 60 calories per serving, with less than 6 grams of sugar or make your own.*

Your favorite veggies. I add ½ cup fresh cut broccoli
½ cup fresh cut cauliflower
½ cup sliced carrots
½ of each: sliced green and yellow peppers
1 small onion, sliced
½ cup mushrooms
½ medium zucchini, chopped

1 garlic clove, chopped
Red pepper flakes (to give it a nice kick)
Salt and pepper to taste
A dash of onion powder
A dash of garlic salt
A sprinkle of oregano
A touch of basil

1) Cook penne as instructed.
2) Spray a large pan with olive oil. Add garlic, onions and mushrooms. Let soften for 5 minutes.
3) Add all your veggies and crisp for approximately 5 minutes.
4) Add tomato sauce and seasonings.
5) Pour in your cooked noodles. Toss and serve.

One Serving

Calories	Carbohydrates	Protein	Fat	Fiber
294	60.4	10.7	2.2	5.9

Peanut Butter Goodness

Serves 2
Make this over ½ cup of cooked brown rice or Shirataki noodles.

1/2 bag frozen raw shrimp, thawed and shelled.
2 Tbsp natural peanut butter
2 Tbsp low-sodium soy sauce
½ green pepper, sliced
½ red pepper, sliced
2 garlic cloves, mashed
½ small onion, sliced
Salt and pepper to taste

1) Spray a large frying pan with olive oil. Sauté garlic and onions.
2) Add shrimp on high and season with salt and pepper. Cook until shrimp begins to change color.
3) Add soy and peanut butter. Coat well. (Peanut butter will want to clump together until it melts.)
4) Add peppers and stir.
5) Add remaining soy and peanut butter.
6) Throw in noodles and blend well.
7) Serve.

Per serving (without rice or noodle)

Calories	Carbohydrates	Protein	Fat	Fiber
202	11.9	17.1	9.1	2.1

Shirataki KD style

Serves 1

This recipe is very similar to the one on the back of the package; I just gave it my own twist. If you're a fan of K.D, you'll love this one.

1 pkg Shirataki fettuccini noodles, rinsed and dried
1 The Laughing Cow light cheese
1 tbsp 0% Greek yogurt
1 tbsp Parmesan cheese
Salt and pepper to taste
1 clove garlic, mashed

1) Place your cleaned noodles, The Laughing Cow cheese, garlic and Greek yogurt in a microwavable bowl.
2) Cook on high for 1 minute. Stir.
3) Sprinkle in Parmesan and cook on high for 1 more minute. Stir.
4) Salt and pepper to taste. Enjoy!

Per serving

Calories	Carbohydrates	Protein	Fat	Fiber
112	8.4	9.1	4.4	4.0

Add 3 ounces cooked white meat chicken to this to make it more of a meal!

Pork Chops

The lone pork chop recipe! I just love it so much I don't make it any other way! But you can stick it on the barbeque and grill it. Pork Chops are actually very lean. They are comparable to chicken.

Pork Chops

Serves 4

4 pork chops, lean & boneless
4 Tbsp honey Dijon mustard
4 tsp maple syrup
Salt and pepper to taste

1) Season chops with salt and pepper on both sides.
2) On each side spread: ½ Tbsp of mustard, ½ tsp maple syrup
3) Heat pan on medium with olive oil spray.
4) Cook marinated chops for about 5-7 minutes on each side.

One 3.5 ounce pork chop

Calories	Carbohydrates	Protein	Fat	Fiber
222	15.7	29.9	4.3	0

Fish & Seafood

It doesn't have to be complicated to be delicious. I have a variety of easy ways I like to cook and eat fish. I've handed over my favorites.

Tuna Bowl on Brown Rice

Sashimi on Brown Rice

Coconut Infused Tuna

Shrimp and Saffron on Brown Rice

Curry Tilapia with Coconut Infused Rice

Fish Tacos

Fish Sticks for Grown Ups

Salmon, My Way!

Creamy Dill Salmon

Tuna Bowl on Brown Rice

Serves 2

1 cup cooked brown rice
* *I like to boil my brown rice in low-sodium chicken broth to give it a light flavor.*
8 ounces sushi grade tuna
1 Tbsp soy sauce
½ Tbsp rice vinegar
½ Tbsp fresh lemon juice
½ tsp sesame oil
1 green onion, diced
2 ounces ripe avocado, cut in cubes (half the fruit)
½ cup shredded lettuce
½ tsp grated ginger (if you don't like ginger, omit)
Sprinkle of toasted sesame seeds

1) Mix wet ingredients and ginger in a bowl.
2) Slice up your tuna into ½-inch cubes.
3) Coat and toss tuna in wet ingredients mixture.
4) When ready to serve, dice your avocado and add it to tuna.
5) Serve over brown rice.
6) Sprinkle toasted sesame and crispy chopped lettuce on top.
7) Feel free to serve with Wasabi.

Calories	Carbohydrates	Protein	Fat	Fiber
324	30.6	30.3	8.7	4.2

Sashimi on Brown Rice

It's as easy at that.

1) Buy some sushi grade fish and serve it on brown rice.
2) Voila!

My favorites are salmon and tuna (also the easiest to get).

Type	Calories	Carbohydrates	Protein	Fat	Fiber
Brown Rice (1/2 cup)	109	22.9	2.3	.8	1.8
Raw Salmon (4 ounces)	161	0	22.5	7.2	0
Raw Tuna (4 ounces)	122	0	26.5	1.1	0

Coconut Infused Tuna

Serves 4

This is a favorite at a little Indonesian restaurant we frequent. My husband loved it so much, he asked me to learn to make it.

1 cup brown rice
2 ¼ cups low-sodium chicken broth

   1) Cook rice as directed using low-sodium chicken broth instead of water. Set aside.

2 cans white albacore tuna in water, drained
2 shallots diced
2 garlic cloves, mashed
1 Tbsp olive oil
1 Tbsp paprika
Dash of cayenne
One low-sodium bouillon cube (beef, chicken or vegetable)
5 Tbsp light coconut milk
1 can (15 oz) whole tomatoes, drained and chopped
Fresh cilantro

   2) Heat oil in a pan on medium. Add shallots and garlic; soften until they begin to caramelize.
   3) Stir in paprika and cayenne to coat shallots.
   4) Add bouillon along with 3 Tbsp of light coconut milk. Stir your mixture until the bouillon dissolves.
   5) Stir in tomatoes and the remaining coconut milk. Mix well.
   6) Add tuna. Bring to a boil and then reduce to low.
   7) Simmer until some of the liquid dissolves. 10-15 minutes.
   8) Top with fresh cilantro.
   9) Serve over brown rice.

One serving and ½ cup of cooked brown rice.

Calories	Carbohydrates	Protein	Fat	Fiber
260	32.2	19.1	6.4	3.5

Shrimp and Brown Rice with Saffron

Serves 4

1 cup brown rice, uncooked
1 package raw shrimp, shelled
1 Tbsp olive oil.
½ bag frozen peas
2 cups low sodium chicken broth
¼ cup low sodium chicken broth
Saffron, large pinch
1 small onion, diced
2 cloves garlic, mashed
Pepper to taste

1) Bring 2 cups chicken broth and 1 cup brown rice to a boil.
2) Reduce to low and simmer until rice is cooked.
3) Sprinkle with ½ tsp Saffron

4) Heat olive oil in a pan on medium/high. Sauté onions and garlic.
5) Add Shrimp and ¼ cup chicken broth.
6) Sprinkle with Saffron (approximately ½-1 tsp).
7) Once shrimp and rice are both cooked, add rice to the shrimp pan and stir in peas.
8) Pepper to taste.

Serve!

Calories	Carbohydrates	Protein	Fat	Fiber
270	28.4	28.9	5	3.5

Curry Tilapia with Coconut Milk Infused Rice

Serves 4

<u>Rice</u>
2 cups light coconut milk
1 cup brown rice
½ cup water
½ tsp salt.

1) Bring coconut milk, water, salt and rice to a boil.
2) Reduce to low and simmer until rice is cooked (covered). Approximately 45 minutes.

<u>Fish</u>
1 tsp olive oil
4 tilapia fillets
2 tsp curry powder
½ tsp ground ginger
½ tsp chili powder
2 garlic cloves, mashed
1 small onion, diced

1) Combine spices in a bowl.
2) Dust tilapia on both sides with spice mixture.
3) Heat a pan on high with 1 tsp olive oil. Sauté onions and garlic.
4) Reduce heat to medium and cook seasoned fillets well on both sides.
5) Serve over coconut infused rice.

One 4 ounce filet and ½ cup of cooked brown rice.

Calories	Carbohydrates	Protein	Fat	Fiber
322	27.6	25.4	11.2	2.6

Fish Tacos

Serves 4

Four tilapia filets
Cajun seasoning

1) Dust filets with Cajun seasoning.
2) Spray olive oil in a pan on medium and cook filets.

Serve Fish with:
Whole grain wraps
Sliced avocado
Diced tomatoes
Shredded cabbage
Light tartar sauce *or* 0% Greek Yogurt (mixed with fresh dill and garlic)

4 Ounce Filet, one Sonoma Wrap, sliced avocado, tomato, cabbage and yogurt.

Calories	Carbohydrates	Protein	Fat	Fiber
206	14.2	29.7	5.6	8.5

* You can also serve with brown rice, pinto or fat-free refried beans!

Fish Sticks For Grown Ups!

Serves 4

16 ounces of white fish like tilapia or halibut
1 ounce ground almond meal
½ cup corn meal
¼ cup whole wheat flour
1 Egg
2 tsp onion powder
2 tsp garlic powder
Salt and pepper to taste

1) Cut fish into 2 or 1 ounce strips.
2) Rinse fish and pat dry fish.
3) On a flat plate – combine Almond Meal, Cornmeal, W.W Flour, and Seasonings.
4) Mix Well.
5) In a bowl, beat egg.
6) Dunk each piece of fish in the egg and then dunk both sides in flour mixture.
7) On the stove top on Medium – spray your pan with Olive oil spray and cook fish until done!
8) Serve with a slice of lemon and a side salad or green vegetable!

Calories	Carbohydrates	Protein	Fat	Fiber
250	18.5	28	7.4	2.7

Salmon, My Way

Serves 4

I used to hate salmon. I thought it was chalky and too fishy. But then "someone" cooked it for me just right! I had been eating it too well done my whole life! So, on that note, do not overcook your salmon.

1 lb salmon (skin on if you can get it)
1 Tbsp of lemon juice
2 garlic cloves, mashed
1 Tbsp brown sugar
3 Tbsp low-sodium soy sauce

1) Place salmon on a tinfoil sheet. Round the edges to make a small wall so that your sauce does not drip out.
2) Squirt your salmon with lemon juice and spread on your mashed garlic.
3) Sprinkle with brown sugar and coat with soy sauce.
4) Place seasoned salmon on covered BBQ on medium/low for approximately 12 minutes.

1 of 4

Calories	Carbohydrates	Protein	Fat	Fiber
252	4.5	25.7	14	.1

Creamy Dill Salmon

Serves 4

1 lb salmon
1 Tbsp of lemon juice
2 garlic cloves, mashed
1 Tbsp 0% Greek style yogurt
1 tsp dried dill
Salt and pepper to taste

1) Place salmon on a large tinfoil sheet.
2) Squirt your salmon with lemon juice.
3) In a small bowl combine yogurt, dill, garlic, salt and pepper.
4) Spread mixture on top of salmon.
5) Cover your salmon with the large tinfoil sheet and seal it so that no air can get out.
6) Cook your salmon pouch on the BBQ on medium/low for 12-15 minutes.

1 of 4

Calories	Carbohydrates	Protein	Fat	Fiber
252	4.5	25.7	14	.1

Salads and Dressings

From bean salad to couscous to good old lettuce—all are quick and easy.
Feel free to toss on a grilled chicken breast, some shrimp or even lean steak.

Bean Salad

Greek Salad Dressing

The Standard Salad Dressing

Twisted Caesar Salad Dressing

Uncle Harvey's Coleslaw

Boo's Chili Lime Quinoa

The Easiest Couscous Ever!

Asiago, Pear and Pine Nut Salad

Jackie's Famous Salad

Simple Salad

My Husbands Favorite Salad

Strawberry, Goat Cheese and Spinach Salad

Bean Salad

Beans are great on a salad, on their own or as a side!

1 cup low-sodium mixed beans, rinsed
1 cup low-sodium garbanzo beans, rinsed
4 celery ribs, diced
½ red pepper, diced
Green onions, chopped
Dried basil to taste (I use 1 ½ Tbsp)
3 Tbsp The Standard Balsamic dressing

1) In a large bowl combine: beans, celery, red pepper, and onions.
2) Coat with 3 Tbsp of dressing and mix well.
3) Add dried basil and toss to coat.
4) Marinate for at least 2 hours—the longer the better.
5) Stir several times over the course of marinating and again before you serve.

One serving. Makes 4 servings.

Calories	Carbohydrates	Protein	Fat	Fiber
174	29	6.3	2.1	6.2

The Standard Salad Dressing

6 Tbsp balsamic vinegar
3 Tbsp olive oil
2 garlic cloves, mashed
1 tsp Honey Dijon mustard
Salt and pepper to taste

1) Combine all ingredients and shake!

1 Tbsp

Calories	Carbohydrates	Protein	Fat	Fiber
40	.3	0	1.1	0

Greek Salad Dressing

3 Tbsp lemon juice
4 tsp red wine vinegar
2 garlic cloves, mashed
2 tsp dried oregano
2 Tbsp canola oil
1 ounce low-fat feta cheese, crumbled
Salt and pepper to taste

1) Combine all ingredients and shake.

1 Tbsp

Calories	Carbohydrates	Protein	Fat	Fiber
42	.6	.2	4.3	.3

Twisted Caesar Salad Dressing

½ cup silken tofu light
¼ cup white vinegar
3 garlic cloves, mashed
1 tsp white horseradish sauce
Salt and pepper to taste
¼ cup grated Parmesan cheese

1 Tbsp

Calories	Carbohydrates	Protein	Fat	Fiber
20	.3	2.5	.3	0

Uncle Harvey's Coleslaw

10 servings. Marinate for at least one day.

1 bag shredded cabbage
2 garlic cloves, mashed
¾ cup white vinegar
¼ cup canola oil (a large portion drips off when you serve)
¼ cup sugar
¼ cup fresh chopped parsley
½ cup shredded carrots
3 green onions, diced

1) In big ziplock bag—mix well: vinegar, oil, sugar and garlic.
2) Add cabbage & carrots. Toss to coat.
3) Add parsley and onions.
4) Marinate overnight in fridge, tossing every so often.
5) Toss before you serve.

Calories	Carbohydrates	Protein	Fat	Fiber
52.7	2.7	.4	2.8	.75

Boo's Chili Lime Quinoa

Serves 4

1 cup cooked quinoa
½ cup black beans, rinsed and drained
2 Tbsp green onions, chopped
1/3 cup canned corn kernels
1 yellow or orange pepper, diced
5 cherry tomatoes (halved)
½ avocado, chopped
½ mango chopped
1 Tbsp fresh cilantro, chopped

Dressing:
1 tsp olive oil
The juice of two fresh limes
Salt & pepper to taste
Cayenne pepper to taste

1) Make dressing. Set aside.
2) Combine 1 cup cooked Quinoa with all the ingredients listed.
3) Dress and toss lightly to coat.

1 Serving

Calories	Carbohydrates	Protein	Fat	Fiber
177	32.5	5.5	2.9	5

The Easiest Couscous Ever

You think couscous is all fancy pants, but it's not!

1) Pick up a box of whole wheat couscous and read the back.
2) It takes 10, yes 10, minutes to make and it tastes delicious, not to mention 7 grams of fiber per serving!
3) Cook it in low-sodium chicken broth instead of water to add more flavor.

*You can follow the recipe on the box or simply add some cranberries and almonds.

Asiago, Pear and Pine Nut Salad

Serves 4

1 bag romaine hearts
½ ounce pine nuts, toasted
½ ounce grated Asiago cheese
1 Bartlett pear, ripe, sliced with skin
2 Tbsp of The Standard Salad Dressing

1) Wash and cut lettuce.
2) Before you serve, add in cheese, pear and nuts.
3) Dress and serve.

Per serving

Calories	Carbohydrates	Protein	Fat	Fiber
89	8.5	2.4	4	2.8

Jackie's Famous Salad

Serves 4

2 bags romaine lettuce
½ cup baby carrots, chopped
2 eggs, diced
1 tomato, sliced
4 celery ribs, chopped
1 ounce low-fat feta cheese, crumbled
3 sliced turkey bacon, chopped

1) Wash and cut lettuce.
2) Throw in all your veggies, cheese, eggs and bacon.
3) Dress with a light creamy dressing.

1 serving without dressing

Calories	Carbohydrates	Protein	Fat	Fiber
120.5	6.9	8.4	6.1	2.7

Simple Salad

Serves 4

1 bag or head butter lettuce
Sliced red, yellow and orange peppers
Cherry tomatoes, halved
Fresh grated Parmesan cheese (1 Tbsp per serving)
2 Tbsp The Standard Salad Dressing

1) Wash and cut lettuce.
2) Throw in your veggies.
3) Dress and top with Parmesan cheese.

1 Serving

Calories	Carbohydrates	Protein	Fat	Fiber
62	5.9	3.4	3.2	1.5

My Husband's Favorite Salad

Serves 4

2 beets, sliced
½ ounce of toasted walnuts
3 artichoke hearts (from can with water)
½ avocado, sliced
1 ounce goat cheese
2 Tbsp The Standard Dressing (or whatever dressing you like)
Bag of leafy greens (your pick!)

1) Wash and cut lettuce.
2) Throw in veggies, cheese, nuts and avocado.
3) Dress and serve!

1 Serving

Calories	Carbohydrates	Protein	Fat	Fiber
131	8.75	4.4	9.4	4.25

Strawberry Goat Cheese and Spinach Salad

Serves 4

1 bag baby spinach
6 or 7 strawberries, sliced
1 oz goat cheese
2 Tbsp The Standard Salad Dressing (or whatever dressing you like)

1) Wash lettuce.
2) Toss in berries and cheese.
3) Dress and serve.

Per Serving

Calories	Carbohydrates	Protein	Fat	Fiber
66.5	5.7	2.8	3.7	1.8

Soups and Side Dishes

Add a side or a soup to whatever you're eating! These are great ways to keep you full without adding crazy amounts of calories.

Kitchen Sink Soup

Mamie's Chicken Soup
Secret Family Recipe!

Chunky Whole Vegetable Soup

Leek and Cauliflower Soup

Chicken and Barley Soup

Zucchini and Basil Soup

Artichoke Hearts

Sweet Potato and Goat Cheese

Sweet Potato Chips

Sweet Potato Fries

Sweet Potato O'Natural

Broccoli and Parmesan

Brussels Sprouts with Currants and Walnuts

Roasted Asparagus

Green Beans with Toasted Almonds

Curry Coconut Corn

Kitchen Sink Soup

It is what it sounds like. Whatever you have in the house, throw it in the pot. This is what mine normally looks like.

1 Tbsp olive oil 2
1 large leeks, diced
2 garlic cloves, minced
1 large carrot
1 parsnips, peeled and cut into chunks
¼-½ head broccoli, cut into pieces
¼-½ head of cauliflower, cut into pieces
1 zucchini
1 cup mushrooms, sliced
1 sweet potato, peeled and chopped
1 small bag frozen green peas
1/2 bag frozen corn nibblets

Low-sodium chicken or vegetable stock (approximately 8 cups)

1) In a large soup pot, heat oil, sauté leeks, garlic and mushrooms.
2) Add the rest of your veggies except peas and corn.
3) Cover your veggies with a low-sodium broth.
4) Bring to a boil and then back down to a simmer on low. Add peas and corn. Cover.

Once the veggies are cooked (about 40 minutes) blend your soup until it has been pureed. This makes a *huge* batch, so I always freeze a bunch for a cold day.

Approximately 1 ½ cups of soup

Calories	Carbohydrates	Protein	Fat	Fiber
71	13	2.8	1.1	2.5

Mamie's Chicken Soup

1 whole raw chicken, quartered, including the neck. It adds a lot of flavor.
4 large carrots, peeled and cut into chunks
2 parsnip, peeled and cut into chunks
2 medium onions, peeled and halved.
3 celery stalks, halved
1 large bunch of dill
Salt and pepper to taste

1) Fill a large pot with water halfway. Bring to a boil and add raw chicken.
2) Skim and strain brownish sludge that forms as chicken begins to boil. 5 minutes.
3) Drop in your veggies and dill.
4) Season with salt.
5) *You can always add more salt after the soup is finished. The salt does brings out the flavor in the soup, however, sodium is NOT your best friend.*

1) Bring to a boil and then simmer on low 1.5 hours, covered with a touch of air peeping through.
2) Allow the soup to cool on your stovetop.
3) Remove all your chicken. Slice up the white meat and put it back in the pot.

To serve and store: pour into refrigerator-safe bowls. Once your soup is cooled completely in the fridge, a hard white layer of fat will form on the top. Remove it and throw it away.
Heat up your soup and enjoy!

1 cup broth with veggies

Calories	Carbohydrates	Protein	Fat	Fiber
117	15.8	6.7	3	1.6

You can add ½ cup of barley to this soup to make it heartier. At the 1 hour mark, pour in ½ cup of pearl barley. Cook for one more hour.

I use half the white meat and half the dark meat to make a chopped chicken salad.

Chunky Whole Veggie Soup

10 servings

1 Tbsp olive oil
3 cups low-sodium vegetable broth
2 baby red potatoes cut into quarters
1 sweet potato, peeled and cut
1 large carrot, peeled and cut
1 medium onion, cut in large chunks
2 garlic cloves, minced
2 leeks, washed and diced (use the whites)
3 celery ribs, cut in pieces
1 15 oz can whole tomatoes, cut in quarters with juice
1 Tbsp tomato paste
1 cup kidney beans, rinsed
Salt and pepper to taste

1) In a large pot, heat olive oil. Sauté leeks, garlic and onions.
2) Add remaining vegetables and pour in vegetable broth, tomato paste and canned tomatoes.
3) Season with salt and pepper.
4) Bring to a boil and then simmer on low until vegetables are cooked. Approximately 30 minutes.

1 Cup

Calories	Carbohydrates	Protein	Fat	Fiber
101	17.2	3.5	2.2	3.8

Leek and Cauliflower Soup

1 Tbsp olive oil
2 large leeks
2 garlic cloves
6 cups chicken stock
1 medium cauliflower head, cut up into chunks
Salt/pepper to taste

1) In a large pot, heat olive oil. Sauté onions and garlic (soften, do not brown).
2) Add stock and cauliflower.
3) Boil for 1 hour.
4) Puree.

1 cup

Calories	Carbohydrates	Protein	Fat	Fiber
54	7	4	1.2	2.1

Chicken Barley Soup

10 cups low sodium chicken broth.
You can use broth from Mamie's chicken soup if you want.
2 raw chicken breast, cut into cubes.
1 onion, diced
2 carrots, cut into cubes
2 celery stalks, cut into cubes
Rutabaga, cut into cubes
Small handful of dill, chopped up
½ cup barley
Pepper to taste

1) In a large pot, bring chicken broth to a boil.
2) Place cubed chicken in broth and cook.
3) Add veggies, dill and parsley.
4) Add barley.
5) Lower to a simmer and cook for 30 – 40 minutes.
6) Pepper to taste.

1 ¼ cup

Calories	Carbohydrates	Protein	Fat	Fiber
102	12	9.5	1	2.3

Zucchini Basil Soup

1 Tbsp olive oil
2 yellow onions
3 large zucchinis, diced
2 garlic cloves
6 cups water
Salt and pepper to taste
Handful of fresh basil leaves

1) In a large pot, heat olive oil. Sauté onions and garlic (soften, do not brown).
2) Add diced zucchinis, sauté for 5 minutes.
3) Add water. Boil on medium until tender.
4) Right before you blend, add a generous handful of basil.
5) Salt and pepper to taste.
6) Blend.

1 cup

Calories	Carbohydrates	Protein	Fat	Fiber
38	5.3	1.2	1.8	1.2

Artichoke Hearts

These are great for an appetizer. It's like the leaves are designed for dipping.

1) Cut the long stem off your artichoke and trim the sharp tips.
2) Place in a boiling pot of water, stem side down. Cover and reduce to low.
3) Simmer for 20-30 minutes depending on the size of your artichoke.
4) When you can easily pluck a leaf, they are done.

Serve along side Hummus or Roasted Red Pepper dip!

Sweet Potato and Goat Cheese

3 medium sweet potatoes
2 Tbsp margarine
2 ounces goat cheese
1 ½ tsp salt
Pepper to taste

1) Peel and cut sweet potatoes. Boil until soft and strain.
2) In a large bowl, mash potatoes, margarine, goat cheese (leave ¼ ounce aside), salt and pepper.
3) Once smooth, place potatoes in serving bowl spread remaining ¼ ounce of goat cheese on top.

These can be made ahead and reheated.

1/8 of Dish

Calories	Carbohydrates	Protein	Fat	Fiber
81	10.2	2.3	3.5	1.4

Sweet Potato Chips

One sweet potato per person. Oven at 450.

When looking for potatoes for this recipe try to buy the ones that are round and long rather than short and fat.

Sweet potatoes
Kosher salt to taste
Pepper to taste
Garlic powder to taste

1) Peel and slice potatoes as thinly as you can, so that you have circular-shaped slices.
2) Spray olive oil on a cookie sheet.
3) Lay the sliced potatoes down so that they each have their own piece of real estate on the cookie sheet.
4) Sprinkle with salt, pepper and garlic powder to taste.
5) Spray the tops of the seasoned potatoes lightly with olive oil, bake in the oven.
6) Flip after 10-12 minutes

* *You have to watch these. Depending on how thin your slices are, they could take 10 minutes or 20 minutes on each side.*

1 medium sweet potato

Calories	Carbohydrates	Protein	Fat	Fiber
124	28.8	2.5	.2	4.1

Sweet Potato Fries

Serves 4. Oven at 425.

4 medium sweet potatoes
Kosher salt to taste
2 cloves garlic, mashed
1 tsp olive oil

1) Cut potatoes into thin sticks so that they resemble French fries.
2) In a large bowl, place already steamed sweet potatoes, oil, garlic and salt. Toss to coat.
3) Spray a lined cookie sheet with olive oil and spread your fries out so that they do not overlap.
4) Bake for 12-15 minutes on each side.

The timing on these can vary depending on the size of your fries. Watch 'em closely!

1 medium sweet potato

Calories	Carbohydrates	Protein	Fat	Fiber
125	26.8	2.1	1.3	3.8

Sweet Potato O'Natural

Oven at 425

Not much of a recipe here.
There is something to be said about the wonderful taste of a baked sweet potato!

1) Poke holes in your potato with a fork.
2) Cover lightly with 1 tsp olive oil and a touch of kosher salt.
3) Place in oven at 425 for 25-30 minutes.

1 medium (5.4 ounce) sweet potato without skin

Calories	Carbohydrates	Protein	Fat	Fiber
115	26.8	2.1	.2	3.8

Broccoli and Parmesan

Yet another no brainer.

Steamed broccoli
1 Tbsp grated Parmesan cheese per person

1) Steam your broccoli.
2) Strain it and place it in serving bowl.
3) Sprinkle with Parmesan cheese and serve.

½ cup steamed broccoli and 1 Tbsp Parmesan cheese

Calories	Carbohydrates	Protein	Fat	Fiber
49	5.8	3.8	1.8	2.6

Brussels Sprouts with Craisins and Walnuts

Serves 8.

2 cups Brussels sprouts
¼ cup toasted walnut pieces
¼ cup dried craisins
1 Tbsp olive oil
1 small onion, diced
2 tsp balsamic vinegar
1 Tbsp honey mustard
Salt and pepper to taste

1) Prepare a pot of boiling water.
2) Wash sprouts, remove stems and slice into strips.

1) Heat olive oil in a pan on medium. Sauté onions until they begin to soften.
1) Pour in balsamic and simmer on low for 5 minutes.
2) Bring heat back up to medium/high and toss in sprouts. Coat.
3) Add dried fruit and walnuts.
4) Season with salt and pepper.
5) Serve.

1 Serving

Calories	Carbohydrates	Protein	Fat	Fiber
83	11	2.4	4.2	1.7

Roasted Asparagus

Oven at 450

1 bunch asparagus
1 tsp olive oil
1 squirt lemon juice
1 ½ tsp kosher salt

1) Wash and trim your asparagus.
2) Place your asparagus on a lined cookie sheet. Lightly drizzle with olive oil, kosher salt and a squeeze of fresh lemon juice.
3) Toss to coat.
4) Bake at 450 for 10-15 minutes.

6 spears

Calories	Carbohydrates	Protein	Fat	Fiber
30	3.7	2.2	1.3	1.8

Green Beans with Toasted Almonds

2 cups green beans (about 50-60 beans)
2 Tbsp toasted almond slices
1 tsp olive oil
Kosher salt to taste

1) Prepare pot of boiling water.
2) Wash and trim green beans.
3) Boil beans for 2-3 minutes. Set aside.

1) Heat olive oil in a pan on medium/high.
2) Sauté beans, toasted almonds and salt.
3) Serve.

¼ of recipe

Calories	Carbohydrates	Protein	Fat	Fiber
45	5.4	1.8	2.4	2.7

Curry Coconut Corn

Corn on the cob
Water
½ cup fat-free milk
Light coconut milk

1) Bring a pot of water and fat-free milk to a boil.
2) Cook corn in boiling water about 10-12 minutes.
3) (You'll know when the corn is done if you poke a kernel with a fork, and it 'pops.')
4) Pour ¼ cup coconut milk on a plate. Roll cooked corn in it.
5) Sprinkle with curry powder and serve.

1 medium piece of corn

Calories	Carbohydrates	Protein	Fat	Fiber
88	18.4	3.2	1.7	3.1

* When boiling corn, always add a large splash of fat-free milk. It really sweetens up your corn.

Dessert Recipes and Quick Sweet Tooth Fix Ideas

*Cut up fresh berries and serve them with low-fat whipped cream!

*½ cup of low-fat ice cream or frozen yogurt.

*Low-fat pudding made with skim milk. You can even buy single servings.

*One serving of graham crackers with 1 Tbsp of Nutella.

*A caramel or chocolate rice cake topped with a handful of melted dark chocolate chips.

*Buy an angel food cake, pile on sliced fresh berries and top with low-fat whip.

A piece of dark chocolate.

Cut up fresh fruit.

Low-fat vanilla yogurt and berries.

Homemade frozen yogurt pops.

Hot cocoa.

Roasted bananas with frozen yogurt.

Fruit salad.

Cheesecake, minus the cake.

Strawberry crumble.

Peanut Butter Chocolate Banana Crunch

Dark chocolate

It's as simple as it sounds. One serving of dark chocolate! Yes, one!
Dark chocolate is good for you, but anything outside of moderation loses its charm very quickly.
A serving of dark chocolate is somewhere in the neighborhood of 220 calories.
Read the label, notice the serving size and follow it.
Try to find a bar that is 70% or higher.

Fresh Fruit

A piece of fresh cut fruit can really settle a sweet tooth. Fruit is nature's candy!
Try a Pink Lady apple, a peach or some blueberries!

Low-Fat Vanilla Yogurt and Berries

It's that simple!

1 serving low-fat vanilla yogurt
Fresh berries

- Please read the nutritional label of the yogurt for calorie counts and serving sizes.

Homemade Frozen Yogurt Pops

Makes 7-8 pops.

1 cup 0% Greek style yogurt
1 ½ cups frozen fruit
1 tsp vanilla extract
2 tsp sugar (or a touch of Agave)

Some Great combos: strawberry, blueberry, raspberry, blackberry
banana, strawberry
pineapple, mango
strawberry, pineapple, mango
banana, pineapple, mango

1) Combine all ingredients in a large bowl and blend to a pulp.
2) Place your mixture into popsicle molds and freeze!

1 Popsicle

Calories	Carbohydrates	Protein	Fat	Fiber
30	4.2	3	0	1

Hot Cocoa

1 cup fat-free milk
1 Tbsp cocoa powder
1 heaping tsp sugar (or a touch of Agave)

1. In a saucepan, bring milk to a boil.
2. Add cocoa powder and sugar until they dissolve.
3. Serve when hot.

Calories	Carbohydrates	Protein	Fat	Fiber
119	19.4	1.4	9.8	1.8

Roasted Bananas with Frozen Yogurt

Serves 4. Broil.

2 cups vanilla frozen yogurt
2 very ripe bananas
4 tsp brown sugar
½ tsp cinnamon

1. Set your oven to broil.
2. Cut 2 very ripe bananas in half, lengthwise.
3. Place bananas on a lined cookie sheet.
4. Sprinkle with brown sugar and cinnamon.
5. Broil for 3-5 minutes.
6. Remove and serve warm over of frozen yogurt.

* *Please see your frozen yogurt container for nutritional information.*

½ warm banana

Calories	Carbohydrates	Protein	Fat	Fiber
57	14.8	.6	.2	1.6

Fruit Salad

Put any fruit into this salad!

2 Tbsp fresh mint leaves, diced
3 or 4 Tbsp soda water

1 cup pineapple, cut into chucks
1 cup watermelon, cut into chucks
1 cup honeydew, cut into chunks
2 kiwis, peeled and cut into chunks
1 cup strawberries, sliced
1 cup blackberries
1 mango, cut into pieces
1 green apple, sliced

1) Toss your fresh mint leaves into your fruit bowl.
2) Drizzle in Soda Water.

1/10th of recipe

Calories	Carbohydrates	Protein	Fat	Fiber
54.5	13.6	.8	.3	2.4

Cheesecake, minus the cake

Fresh Fruit (I use strawberries or blueberries)

4 ounces light cream cheese
½ tsp lemon juice
¼ cup powdered sugar
½ tsp vanilla extract
Graham cracker crumbs

1. In a bowl whip: cream cheese, sugar, lemon juice and vanilla.
2. Top with graham cracker crumbs.
3. Serve as a dip for your fruit!

OR

a) Pour individual bowls of berries and dollop your cream cheese mixture on top.
b) Scoop out the top of your strawberries and fill them with your cream cheese mixture. Sprinkle with a touch of graham cracker crumbs.

1/10th of dip

Calories	Carbohydrates	Protein	Fat	Fiber
38.2	3.4	1.2	2.1	0

Strawberry Crumble

Serves 4

2 pints fresh strawberries, rinsed, dried and sliced.
¼ cup sugar
1 Tbsp lime juice
½ cup low-fat granola

1. Combine fruit, sugar and lime juice in a bowl.
2. Toss to coat.
3. Marinate for 1 hour.

Serve berries in a bowl topped with 2 Tbsp of low-fat granola.

1 of 4

Calories	Carbohydrates	Protein	Fat	Fiber
160	35.5	2.7	2.3	5

Peanut Butter Chocolate Banana Crunch

Serves 1

1tsp natural peanut butter
1 tsp dark chocolate chips (I use Ghiardelli 60% Cacao)
1/2 ounce sliced banana
1 Corn Thin or Rice Cake

1) Melt chocolate chips and P.B together in the microwave for 10 seconds.
2) Stir.
3) Spread onto Corn Thin.
4) Thinly slice banana on top.
5) Finish in the toaster oven or regular oven at 350 until the bananas start to warm!

Calories	Carbohydrates	Protein	Fat	Fiber
86	11.8	2.2	3.9	1.3

References

[1] Scott M. Grundy, MD, PhD. *"Diet Composition. Obesity. Physical Inactivity"* (Primary Prevention of Coronary Heart Disease; Integrating Risk Assessment With Intervention. 1999.)

[2] Cumming S. Apovian CM. Khoadhiar L. *Evidence for Diabetes prevention/Management* (Journal of the American Diabetic Association; Obesity Surgery. 2008.) 40- 44.

[3] U.S. Department of Heath and Human Services. *DASH Eating Plan, Lower your Blood Pressure.* (National Institutes of Health. National Heart, Lung, and Blood Institute. 2006.) 3 - 6.

[4] American Dietetic Association. Fact Sheet: *Step up Nutrition and Health.* ADA. 2007.

[5] U.S. Department of Heath and Human Services. *"Importance of Dietary Guidelines for Heath promotion and disease prevention"* U.S. Department of Agriculture. Dietary Guidelines 2005. heathierus.gov/dietaryguielines.

[6] Olshansky SJ, Passaro DJ, Hershow RC, Layden J, Carnes BA, Brody J, Hayflick L, Butler RN, Allison DB, and Ludwig DS *"A Potential Decline in Life Expectancy in the United States in the 21st Century"* (New England Journal of Medicine. 2005.) 1138-1145

[7] Robert E. Thayer PH.D. *Calm Energy. How People Regulate Mood With Food and Exercise.* 2001. 29-58, 87-111, 155-177

[8] U.S. Department Of Health and Human Services. National Institutes of Health. November 2004 Updated December 2007. NIH Publication No. 07–4098

[9] Natalie Digate Muth M.P.H. , R.D. *Application of Nutrition.* (American Counsel on Exercise Lifestyle and Weight Management Consultant Manual. Second Edition. 2008.) 173

[10] USDA. United States Department of Agriculture. Dietary Guidelines for Americans 2005 www.mypyramid.gov.

[11] Stephen Glass, Gregory Byron Dwyer. *Metabolic Calculations Handbook.* (American College of Sports Medicine. ACS. 2007.) 7

[12] Natalie Digate Muth M.P.H. , R.D. Debra Wein. M.S., R.D., L.D.N., C.S.S.D. *Application of Nutrition. Nutritional Programing.* (American Counsel on Exercise Lifestyle and Weight Management Consultant Manual. Second Edition. 2008.)

[13.] Stephen Glass, Gregory Byron Dwyer. *Metabolic Calculations Handbook.* (American College of Sports Medicine. ACS. 2007.)

[14.] American Dietetic Association. *eatright.org. During National Nutrition Month® 2005 and beyond: To Lose or Manage Your Weight Is All About Calories In, Calories Out.* 01.27.2005

[15.] Journal of American Dietetic Association. *Position of American Dietetic Association. Weight Management. 08/2002.* Volume 102. Number 8. 1145 – 1155

[16.] MD Mifflin, ST St Jeor, LA Hill, BJ Scott, SA Daugherty and Yo Koh. American Journal of Clinical Nutrition. The American Society for Clinical Nutrition, Inc. Nutrition Education and Research Program, University of Nevada School of Medicine, Reno. 1990. Vol 51, 241-247

[17.] Debra Wein, MS., R.D., L.D.N., C.S.S.D., NSCA-CPT. *Nutritional Programming.* (ACE Lifestyle and Weight Management Consultant Manual. 2008) 14-3, 324

[18.] American College of Sports Medicine *Position Stand on Proper and Improper Weight Loss Programs.* 1983. ACSM.

[19.] Meri Raffetto R.D. *How a Very Low Calorie Diet Can Make You Gain Weight.* 2005

[20.] Anthony N. Fabricatore, PhD and Thomas A. Wadden, PhD. *Treatment of Obesity: An overview.* (American Diabetes Association. 2003.) 67-72

[21.] Cedric X, Bryant, Ph.D. Daniel J Green. *Basic Nutrition and Digestion. Macronutrient Structure and Function.* (American Council on Exercise. Lifestyle and Weight Management Consultant Manual Second Edition. 2008) 142- 143

[22.] Mayoclinic.com 2007. 1998-2008 Mayo Foundation for Medical Education and Research (MFMER)

[23.] Micheal A Clark, Scott C Lucett, Rodney J. Corn. *Nutrition. Water.* (National Academy Of Sports Medicine Personal Fitness Training. Third Edition. 2008.) 440 – 442

[24.] Donald S. Roberston M.D, M. Sc. *The Water Heath Report. How Eight Glasses a day keeps the fat off.* Except from *The Snow Bird Diet.* 1986

[25.] F. Batmanghelidj. *Water For Health, For Healing, For Life: You're Not Sick, You're Thirsty*! 2003

[26.] U.S. Department of Health and Human Services. U.S. Department of Agriculture Dietary Guidelines. FDA Nutrition Facts label.

[27.] USDA. United States Department of Agriculture. Dietary Guidelines 2005. mypyramid.gov. Steps to a Healthier you.

[28.] Marlett JA, BcBurney MI, Slavin JL. . *Position of the American Dietetic Association: health implications of dietary fiber.* (American Dietetic Association. 2002.) 933- 1000. * Fiber recommendation 20-35 g/day for healthy adults and age plus.

29. Natalie Digate Muth M.P.H, R.D., Karen Friedmean-Kester M.S., R.D., L.D.N. *Basic Nutrition and digestion. Macronutrient Function and Structure. Carbohydrates.* (American Counsel on Exercise Lifestyle and Weight Management Consultant Manual. Second Edition. 2008.) 136-138

30. Robert Swift, M.D., Ph.D. Dena Davidson, Ph.D. *Alcohol Hangover. Mechanisms and Mediators.* (Alcohol Health and Research World. 1998.) 56

31. Michaele P. Dunlap, Psy.D. Clinical Psychologist. *Biological Impacts Of Alcohol Use: An Overview.*

32. NCADD. National Council on Alcohol and Drug Dependence Inc. Health Check Systems. National Institute of Health. National Institute on Alcohol abuse and Alcoholism. 1997-2008

33. Meri Raffetto R.D., L.D.N. *Weight Fluctuations. Are You Losing Body Fat or Water?* 1997-2008

34. Cythia Sass MPH., R.D. *Weight Fluctuations Explained*! Prevention.2008.

35. Jenna A Bell-Wilson. *Current Concepts in Weight Management.* (American Counsel on Exercise Lifestyle and Weight Management Consultant Manual. Second Edition. 2008.) 187

36. National Dairy Council. *Healthy Weight in Dairy. FAQ.* NDC 1915-2008.

37. Michael A Clark, Scott C Lucett, Rodney J.Corn. *Cardiorespiratory Training Concepts.* (National Academy of Sports Medicine Essentials of Personal Fitness Training. Third Edition. 2008.) 181-183

38. Reviewed By: Harvey Simon, MD, Editor-in-Chief, Associate Professor of Medicine, Harvard Medical School; Physician, Massachusetts General Hospital. David Zieve, MD, MHA, Medical Director, A.D.A.M., Inc. *In Depth from A.D.A.M. Exercise Effects on the Heart.* (New York Times. 3/30/2008)

39. Michael L. Pollock, Ph.D., FACSM (Chairperson), Glenn A. Gaesser, Ph.D., FACSM (Co-chairperson), Janus D. Butcher, M.D., FACSM, Jean-Pierre Després, Ph.D., Rod K. Dishman, Ph.D., FACSM, Barry A. Franklin, Ph.D., FACSM, and Carol Ewing Garber, Ph.D., FACSM 1998. *The Recommended Quantity and Quality of Exercise for Developing and Maintaining Cardiorespiratory and Muscular Fitness, and Flexibility in Healthy Adults.* (American College of Sport Medicine Position Stand – Cardio fitness. 1998.) Volume30, Number 6.

40. James A. Levine, Lorraine M. Lanningham-Foster, Shelly K. McCrady, Alisa C. Krizan, Leslie R. Olson, Paul H. Kane, Michael D. Jensen, Matthew M. Clark. *Interindividual Variation in Posture Allocation: Possible Role in Human Obesity.* (Science. 01/28/2005.) Vol. 307. no. 5709, pp. 584 - 586

41. Presidents Council of Physical Fitness and Sports. *The Blue Program for a Healthier America.* Walking Works. Blue Cross Blue Shield Association. Steps to a Healthier US

42. Michael A Clark, Scott C Lucett, Rodney J.Corn. *Resistance-Training Concepts.* (National Academy of Sports Medicine Essentials of Personal Fitness Training. Third Edition. 271-185